STORYTELLING IN MEDICINE

Throughout our lives, story is the medium each of us uses to make sense of our environment and relationships. Stories provide meaning and context, enriching our experiences and equipping us with a framework to navigate our existence.

This unique, practical book for healthcare trainees, practitioners and educators explores the ideas and practice of narrative and storytelling that lie at the very heart of clinical medicine and the patient 'experience' of care. It shows how story and narrative can be used effectively to help convey concepts such as prognosis and the effect of illness upon life, and to prepare patients and their relatives for difficult and painful news.

Offering a particular insight into communication by and between healthcare professionals, and how it can be refocused and improved, this updated and expanded second edition remains an invaluable teaching aid for educators working in both small and large formats, and for under- and postgraduate students.

STORYTELLING IN MEDICINE

How Narrative Can Improve Practice

Second Edition

Edited by

Colin Robertson
Honorary Professor
Accident and Emergency Medicine and Surgery
University of Edinburgh, UK

Gareth Clegg
Clinical Senior Lecturer and Honorary Consultant
Emergency Medicine
University of Edinburgh, UK

James Huntley
Professor of Paediatric Orthopaedic Surgery
Department of Orthopaedic Surgery
University of Utah
Salt Lake City, Utah, USA

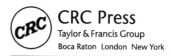

CRC Press
Taylor & Francis Group
Boca Raton London New York

CRC Press is an imprint of the
Taylor & Francis Group, an **informa** business

CONTENTS

CONTRIBUTORS

Gareth Clegg
Senior Clinical Lecturer
University of Edinburgh
and
Honorary Consultant in Emergency Medicine
Royal Infirmary
Edinburgh, UK

Allan Cumming
Emeritus Professor of Medical Education
College of Medicine and Veterinary Medicine
University of Edinburgh
Edinburgh, UK

Graham Easton
Professor of Clinical Communication Skills and Lead for Team Based
    Learning
Queen Mary University of London
Barts and The London School of Medicine and Dentistry
London, UK

James Huntley
Professor of Paediatric Orthopaedic Surgery
Department of Orthopaedic Surgery
University of Utah
Salt Lake City, Utah, USA

Jacques Kerr
Consultant in Emergency Medicine
Royal Victoria Infirmary
Newcastle, UK

Fiona Nicol
Former GP Principal and Trainer
Stockbridge Health Centre
and
Former Honorary Clinical Senior Lecturer
University of Edinburgh
Edinburgh, UK

Sarah Richardson
Specialist Trainee in Emergency Medicine
Edinburgh, UK

Colin Robertson
Honorary Professor of Accident and Emergency Medicine and Surgery
University of Edinburgh
Edinburgh, UK

Joel Symonds
Advanced Practitioner Critical Care
Scottish Ambulance Service
Edinburgh, UK

TO BEGIN AT THE BEGINNING

Colin Robertson and Gareth Clegg

The universe is made of stories, not of atoms.

Muriel Rukeyser

Stories are the most important thing in the world. Without stories, we wouldn't be human beings at all.

Philip Pullman

We swim in a river of change, and we forget its pace. To paraphrase Arthur C Clarke, the Medicine that we practise would be magic to our clinician forebears of even a century ago. Some humility is needed, however. Although frequently forgotten or marginalised, the greatest contributions to human health and well-being come from public health measures: the provision of clean water and sanitation, safe housing, reliable techniques of birth control, and employment. Added to this, immunisation and antibiotic and antiviral drugs have eliminated or dramatically reduced many of the scourges of infectious disease. Consequently, many students or younger clinicians have never seen the common childhood illnesses such as measles, whooping cough or mumps experienced by their parents. Imaging techniques such as CT and MR scanning have transformed both diagnosis and treatment and provide unique insights into physiological processes. Anaesthetic, critical care, innovative surgical techniques and transplantation have opened up treatment possibilities previously considered to be in the realms of science fiction. The potential benefits of genomic diagnosis and treatments, promised for so long, are now becoming a reality,

DOI: 10.1201/9781003409151-1

while controlled trials and evidence-based evaluation are now standard components of healthcare provision. With these extraordinary developments, an observer could be forgiven for considering that satisfaction with the state of medicine should be high. We live longer. In rich countries infant mortality is low. Even with the recent pandemic, death most often results from the diseases of senescence: cardiovascular and cerebrovascular disease, cancer and dementia. So why then are patients, their relatives and the general public so dissatisfied with the provision of medical care? In any survey of patient experience, communication failure is high on the list. Comments often include:

- 'The doctor looked at the screen on the desk, not at me.'
- 'I was talked at, not with.'
- 'I was asked a list of questions and expected to answer Yes or No.'
- 'Nobody listened to my story.'

The societal lockdowns of the COVID-19 pandemic served to exacerbate these concerns. Telephone and audio-video consultations were often used to prevent clinician–patient contact but created new barriers. These consultations work especially poorly if the doctor did not previously know the patient well. Older patients and those with any form of communication difficulty or disability find these contacts inadequate and difficult. Technological problems often aggravate the situation. Dialogue may be disrupted by breakdown or degraded video quality so that subtle nuances of expression are missed, while echoing and latency (the time delay in transmission from one end of the call to the other) lead to stilted conversation (particularly if the delay is greater than 500 ms) producing overlap, interruptions and the need for repetition (Greenhalgh et al., 2016; Wherton et al., 2020).

In the past, and pre-pandemic, clinicians often cited time pressures and targets to excuse difficulties in the consultation. They are feeble, diversionary justifications. Some specialists, focused solely on their organ or disease of interest, fail to see the need to contextualise the patient and their problem. It is worrying to see it stated recently in a major medical journal: 'when physicians take into account the needs and circumstances (that is context) of their patients when planning their care, individualised health care outcomes improve' (Weiner et al., 2013). Really! What did they spend years at medical school doing?

With this background it is unsurprising that 'complementary' therapists are popular and effective with patients (Molassiotis et al., 2005). Homeopathy, aromatherapy, hypnosis, acupuncture, Reiki and massage therapists flourish. 'Conventional' clinicians, educated in randomised clinical trials and an evidence-based approach, may belittle these practitioners and their methods and often highlight potential risks. Nevertheless, many patients say that they achieve benefit even in life-threatening conditions. For some types of cancer, the number of patients using such therapies is up to 50%. Why? The common strand, irrespective of the nature of the therapy, is that these practitioners listen. They give time. They have empathy, acknowledge the patient's fears and communicate hope and support. Even if they cannot cure, they allow the patient to tell their story and, in doing so, restore their sense of identity and individuality (Citrin et al., 2012).

This book is an attempt to redress some aspects that have been trivialised, forgotten or lost in current medical teaching and practice. The advances of the past century are truly extraordinary but, perhaps in the process, we have lost some of the heart of our profession, literally and metaphorically. The arts of storytelling and listening should be central to current medical practice. They can help to re-establish the links with our patients, their relatives, our colleagues and students. They can improve the care and understanding we aim to give.

So this book has some suggestions as to how these techniques can be reintroduced to twenty-first-century medicine. In the telling, there are tales and tasks that may provoke anger, make you laugh and cry or simply ponder and marvel at the human condition: stories of love and loss, life and death, people and places. The contributors are from many backgrounds: primary, secondary and tertiary care doctors, students, academics, actors, artists, and teachers. Most importantly, all are, or have been, patients.

Do not read the book from cover to cover. Dip into it. We suggest that each chapter is seen as a separate facet of the whole picture. In each, the storyteller gives the story with their own voice, character, pace and narrative.

REFERENCES AND FURTHER READING

Citrin D.L., Bloom D.L., Grutsch J.F., Mortensen S.J., Lis C.G. Beliefs and perceptions of women with newly diagnosed breast cancer who refused conventional treatment in favor of alternative therapies. *Oncologist* 2012; *17*(5): 607–12.

Greenhalgh T., Vijayaraghavan S., Wherton J., et al. Virtual online consultations: Advantages and limitations (VOCAL) study. *BMJ Open* 2016; *6*: e009388. http://doi.org.10.1136/bmjopen-2015-009388

Johnsen T.M., Norberg B.L., Kristiansen E., Zanaboni P., Austad B., Krogh F.H., Getz L. Suitability of video consultations during the COVID-19 pandemic lockdown: Cross-sectional survey among Norwegian general practitioners. *J. Med. Internet Res.* 2021 February 8; *23*: e26433.

Molassiotis A., Fernández-Ortega P., Pud D., et al. Use of complementary and alternative medicine in cancer patients: A European survey. *Ann. Oncol.* 2005 April; *16*(4): 655–63.

Weiner S.J., Schwartz A., Sharma G., et al. Patient-centered decision making and health care outcomes. *Ann. Intern. Med.* 2013; *158*: 573–9.

Wherton J., Shaw S., Papoutsi C., et al. Guidance on the introduction and use of video consultations during COVID-19: Important lessons from qualitative research. *BMJ Leader* 2020; *4*: 120–3.

THE POWER OF NARRATIVE AND STORY

Colin Robertson and Gareth Clegg

Without the story – in which everyone living, unborn, and dead partici-pates – men are no more than 'bits of paper blown on the cold wind'.

George Mackay Brown

Narration is as much a part of human nature as breath and the circulation of blood.

A S Byatt

Stories are as essential to human life as the air we breathe; as necessary to our development as food and drink; as critical to our functioning as any of our senses. We are each the author and narrator of our own unique life story. From our earliest days, storytelling has been a fundamental and central part of our lives. Mothers talk and sing to their children, even before they are born. They tell them stories and sing songs. These early 'nursery' rhymes may be simple and naïve, but they become central to the way we form and process ideas as children and adults. They aid our early understanding of the world in which we live and help mould our hopes and fears.

As soon as a child can use language competently, the rate of communication increases dramatically. There can be a true interaction between speaker and listener. This is performed unconsciously, reflexively, without effort, and now we instinctively impose narrative patterns upon the events around us. They provide context and organisation to these events. They provide context, organisation and meaning to our lives. The expanding world of ideas, concepts, objects and their relationships is made intelligible to us through stories.

DOI: 10.1201/9781003409151-2

The way in which our mind processes these stories is not simple. It seems that our brains can produce 'true' stories when they have the appropriate substrate, but have the ability to manufacture 'lies' or fabrications when they don't. There is a compulsion to impose meaning and structure on all information – even random data. This leads to seeing a human face in the shadows on the surface of Mars or Jesus on a piece of toast, examples of a phenomenon the German neurologist Klaus Conrad termed *apophenia* – finding patterns or connections in random or meaningless data. Our hunger for meaningful patterns is not limited to interpretation of sense data, but translates into a genuine hunger for story (see Box 2.1).

BOX 2.1 SHORT FILM

First, watch the short animation film at www.youtube.com/watch?v =VTNmLt7QX8E. Now, in a few words, write down what you saw.

When the makers of the film, Fritz Heider and Marianne Simmel, asked viewers to describe what they saw, most reported stories about the circle and the little triangle being in love, about the big triangle trying to steal away the circle, about the little triangle fighting back, yelling to his love to escape into the house and following her inside where they embraced and lived happily ever after.

The instinctive requirement to resolve uncertainty, randomness and coincidence by enforcing meaning through narrative even works in a retrograde fashion. The Kuleshov effect demonstrates how our brains work to impose a 'back-story' – even when there isn't one. In the early 1900s, Soviet film-maker Lev Kuleshov made a short film in which a shot of an expressionless actor alternated with other apparently random images (a plate of soup, a girl in a coffin, a woman on a divan). Viewers reported that the expression on the actor's face was different each time it appeared, depending on whether he was 'looking at' the soup, the girl in the coffin or the woman on the divan, showing an expression of hunger, grief or desire, respectively. The footage of the actor was actually the same shot each time – the viewers were fabricating their own back-story.

E M Forster, in *Aspects of the Novel*, said that there are only five facts in a human life: birth, food, sleep, love and death. It is therefore unsurprising that the most potent stories reflect these themes, especially the last two. Our stories help us to come to terms with these fundamentals so that we can handle the immensity and chaos of existence. Perhaps it is best to think of the relationship between ourselves and stories as that between fish and water. In the exact same way that water permeates, supports and provides the life-giving medium for fish, so humans cannot live without story.

There is increasing evidence of a structural neurophysiological basis for this; that we are genuinely 'hard-wired' for story. Functional MRI (fMRI) studies in listeners who report a strong understanding of a story show a high degree of 'coupling' with similar events in the storyteller's brain, particularly in the areas of the primary auditory cortex and the temporo-parietal junction where distinction and imagination appear to be processed (Stephens et al., 2010). So, we truly *can* connect with each other. However, this coupling vanishes when participants fail to communicate. This neuronal mirroring may be the basis of our ability to run powerful fictional simulations in our heads and the basis of understanding what is going on in another person's mind.

In general, stories have defined patterns and a predictable set of components. There are three universal elements:

* A character or characters
* The problem
* A resolution of the problem

If any of these is absent from a story we read or are told, we often feel unfulfilled, uncomfortable, somehow cheated. This particularly applies to the resolution phase of the story. Just try telling a 'shaggy dog' story (a story which is long, often with a high level of build-up and complicating action, which ends with an anti-climax or even no ending at all) to a small child to see, and hear, the frustration and exasperation that results. With increasing age and experience, however, most of us come to terms with the reality that not all stories can, or will, have an 'ending'. But that does not necessarily make it easier to accept. For us all, death is the inevitable and final conclusion (see Chapter 12), but interim endings are important and often just as pressing in intensity: will my pain or my symptoms get better? Will I still be able to work and support my family? Could this illness lead to my death?

HELPING THE PATIENT TELL THEIR STORY

A patient's story is their life, intrinsic and inseparable from their being. It defines uniquely their personality and identity. Gaining access to it enables the clinician to reach the nature of their problems, concerns and expectations. It is impossible to overemphasise the importance of the story – or as we would term it medically, the history. All medical teachers exhort their students to 'Listen to the patient. They are telling you the diagnosis.' But many medical students and junior (and senior) doctors continue to ignore this advice. There is a pervasive view that a battery of tests (often complex, expensive, invasive, uncomfortable and time-consuming) will provide the answer. Despite advances in novel imaging techniques, blood tests etc., this is wrong. Frequently this approach confuses and complicates the situation with false-positive and false-negative results and incidental irrelevant findings leading to diagnostic wild-goose chases. In reality, for 70–90% of cases, the correct diagnosis will be made from the history alone (Hampton et al., 1975; Tsukamoto et al., 2012).

BOX 2.2

I need to listen well so that I hear what is not said.

Thuli Madonsela

The best clinicians seem to have an almost instinctive, even magical, ability to obtain an accurate history. Achieving this is central to the practice of clinical medicine and the technique is best learnt by observing skilled practitioners. So how can we, as clinicians, help the patient to give their story? Perhaps the single greatest perceived problem is that of time. Inexperienced clinicians often consider that, with limited time, history taking is best served by a series of directed, usually 'closed' questions (Box 2.3). Sometimes, closed questions are indeed necessary, but usually only later in the consultation. Initially, open questions with an encouraging comment or prompt such as 'And then?' or 'Uh-huh' are the secret to helping the patient give their story. Remember the process of watching a play or film. There is no point in interrupting or fast-forwarding before the 'Character(s)' and the 'Problem' have been developed – the denouement and its resolution will hopefully come from you later.

BOX 2.3 OPEN AND CLOSED QUESTIONS

- **Open questions** encourage the patient to talk. They commonly start with a word such as 'What' or 'Where', or a phrase: 'Please tell me more about ...'. They are crucial early in the consultation when you are trying to find out what is going on and encouraging the patient to talk.

- **Closed questions** seek specific information, usually as part of a systemic enquiry: Do you have a cough? Do you have heartburn? and so on. They invite monosyllabic 'Yes' or 'No' answers and so obstruct the flow of the patient's story.

(Adapted from Macleod's *Clinical Examination*, 13th edition, p. 7)

For years, traditional medical history taking has followed a sequential and set pattern of questioning. This format has been promoted by the increasing use of structured electronic records, checklists and forms. The conventional sequence of questioning is:

- History of presenting complaint
- Past medical history
- Drug history and allergies
- Family history
- Social history
- Systemic enquiry of systems – cardiovascular, respiratory, urinary etc.
- Is there anything else we haven't covered?

But much of a patient's problem is inextricably linked to their personal situation and this technique may be outmoded. Barry Wu from Yale University suggests that reversing the order of questions (see following) takes no longer and helps to put the patient's story into context. Asking about the social and family history first may seem counterintuitive, but it conveys your interest in the patient as an individual, fosters the patient–doctor relationship and your understanding of their problem(s). It may give crucial clues as to the nature of the problem even before the presenting complaint is approached, for example in relation to their occupation, family dynamics etc. Provided the process is explained carefully beforehand, the patient will feel that they are an individual, not simply viewed as a case of chest pain or breathlessness. As Sir William Osler said, 'The good physician treats the disease; the great physician treats the patient who has the disease.'

REVERSING THE ORDER OF HISTORY TAKING

- Social history
- Family history
- Drug history and allergies
- Past medical history
- History of presenting complaint
- Systemic enquiry of systems – cardiovascular, respiratory etc.
- Is there anything else we haven't covered?

(Adapted from Wu, 2013)

LISTEN FIRST, LISTEN SECOND

Every storyteller wants an attentive, interested audience whose participation assists and does not interrupt or inhibit the narrative flow. In real life, however, it seems that this rarely happens. Basically, we fail to listen. Studies of recorded doctor–patient interviews show that less than a quarter of patients were allowed to complete even their opening statement of concerns. The mean time to interruption was 12 seconds in one study and 18 seconds in another! In over two-thirds of the consultations, the doctor then interrupted with questions directed towards a specific concern (closed questions). Worryingly, in addition, elements of sexism intrude: doctors (both male and female) are more likely to interrupt a female patient than a male one (Rhoades et al., 2001; Beckman & Frankel, 1984).

The skills needed to recognise, absorb and interpret a patient's story have been called 'narrative competence' (Charon, 2000, 2004; Divinsky, 2007). Narrative competence, in some ways, necessitates a return to some of our childhood attitudes and experiences: listening carefully to ensure that you miss nothing of the story's structure and perspective and that all the insinuations and metaphors are identified; the need for creativity and curiosity to interpret the tale and conceive different endings; the emotional or affective talent to appreciate the patient's mood and nature.

Some people seem to have these talents innately. There are charismatic individuals who, when you meet, have the ability to make you feel that you are, at that moment, the most important person in their life. Without being obtrusive, they hang on to your every word. Politicians cultivate these skills, and proficiency in these techniques can be learned. In the UK and Europe, although there are some notable exceptions, medical education has lagged behind in this area. Many senior clinicians still view the ideas as woolly or self-indulgent 'soft skills'. By contrast, in North America teaching in narrative competence is increasingly part of mainstream medical teaching.

BOX 2.4 HOW TO IMPROVE YOUR NARRATIVE COMPETENCE

* Read 'good' fiction. If you are in any doubt as to what is 'good', start with some of the '100 Best Books' on websites such as the BBC, *Guardian*, *Telegraph* etc.). When we read, we 'experience' and 'feel' the struggle of the protagonist.
* Write about your experiences – medical and personal. If you can, share your writing with others. The simple act of writing helps to formulate and crystallise your views. Review, after a period of time, what you have written. Is it stilted, naïve, even wrong?
* Read patients' stories. The personal accounts in, for example, the *BMJ* or at www.mayoclinic.org/patient-stories are often deeply moving. In a few words, they give extraordinary insight into being a patient, their illnesses and interactions with the medical profession.
* Take time to reflect on these things.

The single greatest attribute and the best chance for you to help your patient is your ability to listen. However, listening is *not* merely sitting passively; it involves active participation. Active listening involves the other senses as well as your ears. Here, regrettably, technology intrudes. You may think that you can simultaneously listen competently while entering information on a screen. You can't. Listen first and type, or write, afterwards.

Inhibiting the patient's story is all too easy. Patients may have communication difficulties or be intimidated by the environment or by aspects of social stigma. So be aware particularly of non-verbal pointers such as facial expression and body language that often complement or highlight the verbal story.

Physical factors such as sitting behind a computer screen, telephone calls, noisy environments or if the discussion may be overheard (curtains and screens never offer privacy) will prevent the patient from telling their story. So too may your personality and body language. Your nature, your ego, your beliefs, code of ethics or prejudices should never obstruct the patient's narrative.

Fundamentally, you have to be interested in the person in front of you. We all have 'off-days', but if you are not interested in your patients perhaps you should ask yourself: 'Is *clinical* medicine really for me?' Implicit in this interest is empathy. Crucially, empathy is *not* the same as sympathy, an expression of sorrow. Empathy communicates to your patient that you understand and appreciate at least some of what they are experiencing. One way of achieving this is to imagine that their story is yours. How would you feel, behave and react in their position or situation? (Table 2.1).

Obtaining the story begins the patient–doctor interaction. Subsequently, at various stages you will need to communicate with the patient and, often, their family. This may be about what is going to happen next; for example, further investigations, what treatment is proposed, its effects and the likely outcome. We often find this process uncomfortable. We train as scientists and are in comfortable, familiar territory dealing with facts and figures, physiology and pathology. But we are much less happy with communicating uncertainty and dealing with emotion. What are realistic goals? Can we give a true appreciation of the risks and benefits implicit in our therapeutic plan?

Many of these inadequacies relate to deficiencies in our education. We learn and are regularly tested on facts, data interpretation and practical techniques. Increasingly, communication skills are tested in examinations, often with actors playing the part of patients or relatives. What is more difficult to impart is the wisdom and empathy as to how best to apply this precious knowledge to an individual patient facing you. The process is also hampered by a natural wish to be perceived by your patient as an 'all-knowing' healer with a vast, powerful store of modern diagnostic and therapeutic aids at your fingertips. Together, these factors can produce a refuge in aloofness or distance, the 'glass wall approach'; others may adopt the attitude that 'I have the knowledge and the power, I must be right.' In many clinics, hospitals and lecture rooms the cult of the 'doctor as God' persists.

An ability to use a narrative or story format can solve or prevent many of these difficulties. It can give unique communication benefits,

Table 2.1 Helping the patient tell their story

- Try to appear unhurried and convey that you have time for them.
- Always start with 'open' questions.
- Let them tell their own story – not what you want to hear.
- Do not interrupt. A short silence will often prompt the patient better than you asking another question.
- Do you really understand the story the patient is telling you? If necessary, ask them to clarify what they mean.
- Find out about your patient as an individual.
- Acknowledge their emotions.
- Find out about their ideas, concerns and expectations (ICE).

enabling you to communicate and explain concepts which otherwise would be difficult or impossible (Charon, 2004). In many ways the technique mirrors the process used to enable the patient to tell their story. However, there are some important additional points:

• Speak slowly and clearly
• Keep your sentences short
• Use language and words that are fully understood by the patient
• Use your body language and non-verbal communication to aid your technique
• Allow time for the message to 'get through'

Any storyteller who uses jargon, technical terms or euphemisms is unpopular. If you are in any doubt, ask the patient what they understand by a term you have used. Even if they understand the words, do they appreciate the implications of what you have said? For example, many patients still believe the word 'cancer' automatically means a death sentence when, in reality, the form of cancer they have may be curable, or at least not imminently fatal. Simple words can later, if necessary, be expanded in complexity as the patient's comprehension increases: 'There is a growth in your bowel ... It is a form of cancer ... However, we can treat this type of cancer with ...'

Although language is the primary mechanism of communication, some patients may be inarticulate. This may be because they don't know the words to use, or they have a desire not to 'complain'. This is particularly the case with elderly patients. Even if the patient cannot find the right words, they may be able to indicate their feelings or situation in some other way. Non-verbal approaches such as drawings or paintings may be brought to the consultation. Drawing and painting can give especially poignant story representations. Look at the sequence of paintings produced by artist John Bellany (1942–2013) before, during and after his liver transplant – the colours alone provide clues as to his state. In a paper titled 'Developing narrative competence in students', Louise Younie published a powerful painting by one of her students which encapsulates her interaction with a middle-aged woman with a depressive illness (Younie, 2009). For the less artistic, even a simple line can tell the story. In his master's thesis (which incidentally was rejected!) the writer Kurt Vonnegut proposed that a character in a story, and the story itself, could be formulated in graphic form – giving a pictorial representation of their state (Figure 2.1).

Finally, to ensure that the patient and/or their relative fully grasps the story you have given them, get them to précis the information. Particularly for complex situations, some clinicians give a recording

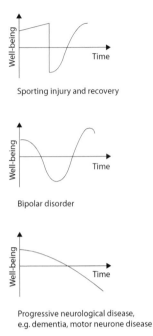

Figure 2.1 Some shapes of stories.

of the consultation to the patient. This enables them to replay and assimilate the information at leisure.

OUR STORY

Stories seem to be essential to give structure to human life. They impose meaning on the empirical data of our existence to form a kind of 'cognitive script' – a framework within which we can ask and interpret some of life's central questions: Where have we come from? Why am I the way I am? Where am I going? From an evolutionary perspective, what is it about story which has made it so pervasive and necessary? Is our need for narrative an evolutionary adaptation or simply a carry-over or side effect? The evolutionary psychologist Jonathan Gottschall poses the question this way: 'Evolution is ruthlessly utilitarian. How has the seeming luxury of fiction *not* been eliminated from human life?' (Gottschall, 2012).

Several possibilities exist: stories may be a kind of mating ritual – a cognitive 'peacocking' to attract sexual partners. Perhaps they constitute a 'cognitive play' analogous to the physical rough and tumble of children, acting as a workout for our mental muscles. Or are stories a low-cost source of vicarious experience – a kind of 'mental holodeck' or flight simulator which allows us mental thrills without the cost of earning the stimulating neurochemicals the hard way in the 'real world', but which still equip us for future life experiences? Our brains may be innately wired for stories, but they are generated within the confines of our own cultural context. Our stories define who we are, and, in turn, we are created by the stories 'allowed' in our culture: 'stories are working on us all the time, reshaping us in the way that flowing water gradually reshapes a rock' (Gottschall, 2012). Our emotional state has a huge impact on this process. Successful people's stories commonly contain themes of redemption. For them, negative events, failure, disruption, loss or pain, tend to transition into positive outcomes. Analysis of self-reported life stories shows that highly productive people have twice as much of this redemptive content as the rest of us.

Naturally, our life stories constantly evolve. As we get older, the complexity of character, themes and drama increases; the process seems to peak in middle age, after which our stories tend to simplify again, but also become more positive. Memory translates our past life into the form of a novel with 'chapters' based on significant life events. We can imagine our future as chapters that have yet to be read. If you wish to put yourself into some form of structure or context, consider that the 'average' human lives for about 4,000 weeks. How many have already passed you by?

Reflecting on the big questions about who we are and our purpose in life is crucial in shaping narrative identity. The stories that these questions provoke can help us to take control over our life; they can rewire our brains in positive ways. In medicine we are shepherded by the demands of our education and work-life at rates that often preclude sustained personal reflection. When we are brought to a standstill, often by some particularly difficult life event, the necessity to find a context for what is happening in our personal or professional life may painfully expose the superficiality of our self-understanding. Then we need to ask: 'Am I the victim of my story or the master of my destiny?'

REFERENCES AND FURTHER READING

Arbesman S. *The half-life of facts: Why everything we know has an expiration date.* New York: Penguin Books; 2013.

Beckman H.B., Frankel R.M. The effect of physician behavior on the collection of data. *Ann. Intern. Med.* 1984; *101*: 692–6.

Charon R. Literature and medicine: origins and destinies. *Acad. Med.* 2000; *75*: 23–7.

Charon R. Narrative and medicine. *NEJM.* 2004; *350*: 862–4.

Cron L. *Wired for story: The writer's guide to using brain science to hook readers from the very first sentence.* Berkeley, CA: Ten Speed Press; 2012.

Divinsky M. Stories for life: introduction to narrative medicine. *Can. Fam. Phys.* 2007; *53*: 203–5.

Evans D. *Risk intelligence: How to live with uncertainty.* New York: Simon and Schuster; 2012.

Frank A.W. *Letting stories breathe: A socio-narratology.* Chicago, IL: University of Chicago Press; 2010.

Geary J. *I is an other: The secret life of metaphor and how it shapes the way we see the world.* New York: HarperCollins; 2011.

Gottschall J. *The storytelling animal: How stories make us human.* New York: Houghton Mifflin Harcourt; 2012.

Hampton J.R., Harrison M.J.G., Mitchell J.R.A. et al. Relative contributions of history-taking, physical examination, and laboratory investigation to diagnosis and management of medical outpatients. *BMJ.* 1975; *2*: 486–9.

Rhoades D.R., McFarland K.F., Holmes Finch W. et al. Speaking and interruptions during primary care office visits. *Fam. Med.* 2001; *33*: 528–32.

Sachs J. *Winning the story wars: Why those who tell – And live – The best stories will rule the future.* Boston, MA: Harvard Business Review Press; 2013.

Smith R. Thoughts for new medical students at a new medical school. *BMJ.* 2003; *327*: 1430–3.

Spiro H., McCrea Curnen M.G., Peschel E., et al. *Empathy and the practice of medicine: Beyond pills and the scalpel.* New Haven, CT, and London: Yale University Press; 1996.

Stephens G.J., Silbert L.J., Hasson U. Speaker-listener neural coupling underlies successful communication. *Proc. Nat. Acad. Sci. USA.* 2010; *107*(14): 425–30.

Tsukamoto T., Ohira Y., Noda K. et al. The contribution of the medical history for the diagnosis of simulated cases by medical students. *Int. J. Med. Educ.* 2012; *3*: 78–82.

Wu B. History taking in reverse: beginning with the social history. *Consultant.* 2013; *53*: 34–6.

Younie L. Developing narrative competence in students. *Med. Humanit.* 2009; *35*: 54.

STORIES IN THE CONSULTATION

Graham Easton

Narrative medicine has revolutionised our thinking in many aspects of healthcare, but what does it mean for the doctor or healthcare professional in their daily work seeing patients? In this chapter I explore how the narrative revolution goes to the very heart of medicine – its central act, the consultation between doctor and patient. I will set out how a narrative understanding of what goes on in consultations can help you and your patients, show you some skills to help you put narrative theory into practice and introduce a narrative framework of the consultation to help you make sense of the stories that your patients are trying to tell.

WHY STORIES ARE IMPORTANT IN THE CONSULTATION

Narrative medicine hinges on the idea that patients (and their doctors) make sense of health and illness by constructing stories (or narratives – I'll use the terms interchangeably here). In our urge to impose some sort of understandable order on the chaos of our lives, we instinctively turn to narrative structures. We make sense of new experiences by weaving new stories into old ones – meaningful reality becomes a sort of tapestry of language that is continually being woven (Launer, 2002).

Using this narrative perspective, the consultation can be understood in terms of the stories that patients and doctors are trying to tell. For the consultation, this means that the conversations you have with your patients aren't just stories about an objective reality of illness; they can create a new reality (Launer, 2002). The health professional becomes someone who pays attention to patients' stories and can help

DOI: 10.1201/9781003409151-3

patients to create helpful, satisfactory and meaningful stories about illness and health. The doctor becomes a co-creator of stories with the patient. Medicine becomes more about helping patients to tell stories that 'fit', or even, as in mental healthcare, helping people to develop different stories about themselves (Launer, 2002).

Of course, telling and listening to stories is not all a doctor is doing – he or she still needs to be an expert: understand what's wrong, make diagnoses, order tests and do procedures for example. But the idea is that all this goes on within a meshwork of stories.

WHAT STORIES ARE TOLD IN THE CONSULTATION?

The consultation is brimming with stories (Figure 3.1). You could think of it as a 'story stew'. There may be many different stories

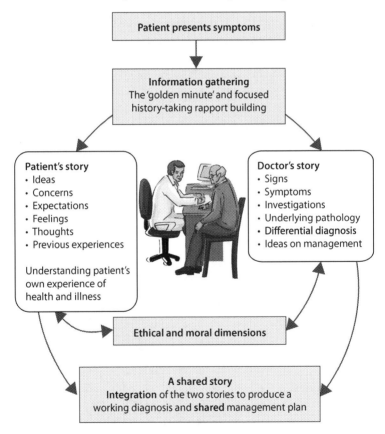

Figure 3.1 The three main stories in the consultation. (Adapted from Stewart & Roter, 1989.)

floating about in this stew, but for simplicity, it helps to focus on three especially juicy story chunks. These are the patient's story (or stories), the doctor's story and the shared story they must create together. If you see patients, you will be used to hearing their stories. Some are just snippets ('My legs are killing me doc … I've reached the end of my tether'), and others are much fuller stories with lots of detail and a clear plot ('It all started last Tuesday when I was doing the gardening …'). Patients may have several stories to tell, or just one. They may be complete or unfinished. They may change over time, and vary according to who is listening. But however they present themselves, these stories or narratives are how patients choose to tell you about their illnesses – they are usually personal and add important context and meaning for the patient which they want to share with you. A diagnosis or treatment that fails to take notice of that context, or that doesn't easily weave into the patient's existing narrative understanding, is unlikely to be meaningful or helpful for the patient. It's also less likely to be accurate – as Sir William Osler is supposed to have said: 'Listen to your patient – he is telling you the diagnosis.' And as Stewart and colleagues say, the greatest single problem in clinical interviewing is the failure to let the patient tell their story (Stewart et al., 1995). So as doctors we need to pay close attention to these patient stories, and become experts in helping patients to tell the stories they need to tell.

But it is not just your patient who is telling stories, or using narrative structures. You, the professional, have your own story to 'tell'. This is the professional account we have all been trained to gather about the patient since medical school. It is also the narrative genre we all use to communicate with each other about our patients. If you are an experienced clinician, this story is probably very familiar to you; you've heard it many times before. It's the one about the patient's presenting complaint, their past medical history, their family and social history, their medication history, your examination findings, your investigations, your differential diagnosis and your management plan.

This medical narrative account is fantastically efficient at gathering relevant information to guide diagnoses and treatments. But while the medical case history is a proven tool for tackling the question 'What is wrong with this person?', it risks dehumanising patients by stripping the objective, factual and scientific details of disease from an individual's narration of suffering (Sobel, 2000). To put it another way, in a patient's story, the protagonist or lead character is usually the patient; but in a doctor's story, the protagonist is often the body or the illness. The doctor's story can rip the soul from the patient's experience. So, in narrative terms, the doctor must attempt a difficult juggling act here, creating a vital professional account while at the same time paying attention to the patient's personal story. It can sometimes feel like rubbing your head while patting your stomach at the same time. The danger is that the professional story often drowns out the patient's one. As the clock ticks by in a busy clinic, we are all tempted to concentrate on telling our professional story at the expense of the patient's personal one.

The third juicy chunk of story stew in a consultation is the shared story that the patient and doctor are trying to create together. In a sense it isn't a separate story at all; it's really an amalgam of the patient's and doctor's stories. Storytelling is an interactive social activity, a co-creation between a narrator and a listener. The clinical task is accomplished through the interplay of two voices in a discourse – as Mishler puts it, the voice of medicine and the voice of the patient's 'lifeworld' (Mishler, 1984). Your challenge is to somehow create together a story that is acceptable – and meaningful – for both of you, and that satisfies both your professional needs and your patient's personal needs. In practical terms, this co-creation means involving the patient in decision making, negotiating a shared management plan and often redrawing the balance of power in the consultation so that it becomes more patient-centred.

HOW THINKING ABOUT STORIES CAN HELP YOU AND YOUR PATIENTS

So why should you bother with these narrative ideas about the consultation? How could it help you or your patients?

Perhaps the most obvious benefit is that a narrative perspective simply offers another way to think about the consultation, in particular to focus on the patient's story, and to bring to the foreground the process of shared decision making and management planning. It can also act as a constant reminder of the power balance between you and your patient – whose story is coming over loudest and clearest? It's also another tool we can use in training and to analyse our consultations, particularly when they seem to go wrong.

As Launer suggests, the narrative paradigm can also reinvigorate our professional curiosity and enrich our daily work by drawing attention to the huge variety of stories, beliefs and cultures we hear every day. And seeing stories as powerful agents of change, in themselves, can relieve us of the pressure we can feel to 'do something medical' every time we are faced with a patient's problem (Launer, 2002).

Being patient-centred involves having the patient's story at the heart of the consultation: listening to it attentively, understanding it and taking account of it. Research suggests that patient-centred consultations correlate with clinical measures such as prescribing the right treatments, taking a reliable history and giving appropriate information (Roter & Hall, 2006). We also know that effective communication leads to fewer investigations and referrals and less need for follow-up appointments (Little et al., 2001), and Levinson et al. have shown that doctors who negotiate the structure and expectations of the consultation explicitly with the patient are less likely to be sued (Levinson, 1994).

A patient-centred approach is also key in empathising with patients: seeing their perspective and understanding some of the emotions they feel. Patients seem to want empathic doctors looking after them (Halpern, 2003). There is also growing evidence that, by some measures, empathy can enhance the doctor–patient relationship, improve both patient and doctor satisfaction (Mercer & Reynolds, 2002) and even improve clinical outcomes, for example in diabetic patients (Hojat et al., 2011).

Yet we also know that, despite all this evidence, doctors tend to interrupt patients' stories after only about 20 seconds (Beckman & Frankel, 1984; Marvel et al., 1999). When patients' narratives are interrupted, the consultation becomes less patient-centred, and patients tend to start telling their narratives all over again, taking even more time. Understanding how patients tell stories and what you can do to help them is likely to improve patient-centeredness and empathy.

The narrative approach also highlights the collaborative nature of consultations – the central task of co-creating an acceptable story between patient and doctor. There is growing evidence in favour of shared decision making in the consultation (De Silva, 2012):

- Patients are more satisfied with their care
- Patients are better informed
- Patients are more confident in their decisions
- Patients are more actively involved in their care
- Patients may be more likely to adhere to their chosen treatment
- There are no apparent adverse effects on health outcomes
- There is little robust evidence of benefit in health outcomes (not enough long-term studies yet)

And yet the evidence from patient experience surveys suggests that while doctors might think they share decision making with patients, they rarely do (Elwyn et al., 2012). Perhaps a narrative approach could help.

NARRATIVE CONSULTATION SKILLS FOR DOCTORS

So how can doctors and health professionals make practical use of this narrative understanding of the consultation?

For a start, many of the existing communication skills and consultation models we are taught can be understood in terms of how doctors can help patients to tell their stories, and how you can create a shared story with your patient. Here are a few key examples.

OPEN QUESTIONS

We are trained to use open questions, which don't demand a yes or no answer, at the beginning of consultations (Silverman et al., 1998). While closed questions (which invite specific answers, often yes or no) are useful for covering specific clinical issues (alarm symptoms, review of systems or allergies for example), they can close down the patient's story. Open questions, on the other hand, encourage patients to tell the story they want to tell: to start the way they want, and to steer the story in the direction they want it to go.

Even the questions we use to begin a consultation can shape the story the patient tells. For example, I often say, 'Good morning Mr XXX. How can I help you today?' It usually works fine, and the patient tells me what they want me to hear. But on a couple of occasions, patients have looked at me with a puzzled expression, and have stopped in their tracks before they have even got going. The patient's response was something like: 'I hadn't really thought about how you could *help* me. I was going to tell you what's been happening and then take it from there.' The way I worded my invitation to the patient steered him in a direction he wasn't expecting to go, and completely threw him. It was me – not the patient – in the driving seat. So we should try to let the patient take the steering wheel, by thinking carefully about the sorts of questions we ask and how they can constrain or free up patients in their storytelling.

· You might reasonably be worried that by encouraging patients to tell their stories – for example by asking open questions – you risk opening 'a can of worms'. Your patients will just talk more and more, and your busy clinic will run later and later. But the evidence suggests that doesn't happen. In one study, if left uninterrupted, most patients stopped talking in less than 45 seconds, and even the most talkative had wound up by 2½ minutes (Beckman & Frankel, 1984).

ACTIVE LISTENING

Active listening skills include encouraging body language and speech (for example paralanguage such as 'Mmm', 'Uh-huh', 'I see', or 'Go on …'), making eye contact, head nodding and silence. These are the skills you probably use naturally when you listen to friends' stories. You lean forward, you focus on the storyteller, you might even nod or make encouraging noises. Above all, you let them speak when they have a story to tell (what's called 'extended turn-taking' in narrative circles). Showing empathy – often most authentic through body language (a concerned frown, or appropriate touch) rather than specific words ('That must have been awful for you') – can be a very effective way to show someone that you are fully engaged with their story.

IDEAS, CONCERNS AND EXPECTATIONS (ICE)

This is the Holy Trinity of patient-centred consultations: it is almost a medical cliché now, but eliciting the patient's ideas, concerns and expectations (ICE) remains a pivotal consultation skill (Pendleton et al., 2003). In story terms, these are often bits of the story that patients leave out, either deliberately or subconsciously. The skills of establishing what the patient thinks might be going on, what their worries are and what they hope might happen, are skills in helping the patient tell important parts of their story. This is the personal, emotional and contextual information that will help you as a doctor to co-create a final story that resonates with the patient. Establishing the patient's concerns early on can also avoid last-minute concerns arising much later in the consultation (Marvel et al., 1999).

SUMMARISING

Summarising is a useful tool in storytelling. It shows the narrator (patient) that you have been listening, and it allows you both to check that you are happy with the story so far. Doctors often think summarising is just for the end of a consultation – but the maxim 'Summarise early and often' is a good one. And think about letting the patient summarise sometimes; it challenges the default power balance in the consultation.

SIGNPOSTING

Signposting (telling the patient clearly where you are going next in the consultation) is a narrative skill. It's a device for navigating the patient through the professional story that you want to tell, which is an unfamiliar landscape for most patients. You might use signposting to signal a change from open questioning to more focused or closed questioning. For example, 'Thank you. Now I'd like to ask a few very specific questions to help me find out what's going on.

Would that be alright with you?' This is really a courteous way to ask permission to focus on your professional story now. If this gear change in the consultation is not introduced carefully and with an explanation, it can seem dominating, rude and often confusing (for example, when you suddenly start asking about a patient's sexual history when they can't see an obvious link with their skin complaint).

CUES

During consultations patients give out signals, or cues, that can be both verbal and non-verbal. They can be subtle; but they can also be very significant moments in a consultation and as doctors we don't want to miss them. It can be helpful to acknowledge these cues when you notice them because they can lead to a crucial part of the patient's unfolding story which may never have been told. An example of a cue might be a patient repeating a word like 'worried' or 'stressed' more than once. They may not quite know how to broach their concern that they have a stress-related illness. In this instance, you could say, 'I notice you've said the word "stress" a few times now. Is that something that you're concerned about?'

The stories patients tell are not always said 'out loud'; many cues are non-verbal. In narrative terms, being attentive to cues is all about tuning into the subtext of the patient's story, the white spaces that can often say as much as the spoken story itself. For example, when a patient spends a moment gazing into space (what Neighbour calls the internal search), you might give him space to search, and then ask whether he wants to mention what he was thinking about just then (Neighbour, 2004). For the patient who seems close to tears, you might say, 'I noticed you seemed a little upset when we were discussing XYZ ... would you like to talk about that?'

All these skills can be framed in terms of helping patients tell their stories, paying close attention to their stories and co-creating constructive stories with them. But there have been attempts to focus more specifically on the benefits of a narrative perspective on the consultation. In particular, John Launer, a GP and family therapist, has described a narrative-based model of consulting.

Launer describes a useful conceptual framework for thinking about a narrative-based approach, called the seven Cs (Launer, 2002), as follows.

- **Conversations**: Conversations don't just describe reality; they can create it. You can think of conversations as interventions in their own right. Launer and his team teach skills for 'conversations inviting change': exploring connections, differences, new options and new realities.
- **Curiosity**: With curiosity you can invite patients to reframe/reconstruct their stories. Curiosity is neutral – to people, blame, interpretations, facts.
- **Contexts**: This is where your curiosity should be focused: families (genograms can be helpful triggers), history, beliefs, values. What is your context? What do patients expect of you?
- **Circularity**: The idea here is to get away from the linear concept of cause and effect, and unchangeable problems, and instead help the patient to focus on meanings. This might involve using circular questions (perhaps based on the words that patients use, and using questions which promote a descriptive rather than explanatory world view).
- **Co-construction**: What you are trying to do with the patient is to create a story that makes better sense for people of what they are going through, a better reality than the present one.
- **Caution**: Don't be unrealistic about your own resources or cover up for the lack of others. Don't upset patients or get scared.
- **Care**: For Launer, this is central to the whole process as, without it, nothing else works.

Launer also describes some very useful techniques for helping to understand patients' stories (Launer, 2002). This is based on the idea of interventive interviewing, an idea first postulated by the Milan team of family therapists in the 1980s, and further developed by Canadian psychologist Karl Tomm. Instead of the term 'interventive interviewing', Launer prefers 'conversations inviting change'. The skills involve moving between four main types of questions: linear questions (factual questions, like those asked in a medical clerking); strategic questions (leading questions designed to nudge people in particular directions, e.g. 'Why don't you try …?'); circular questions (see earlier – questions that draw attention to the way the world operates on circular rather than linear principles); and reflective questions (particular kinds of circular questions aimed to invite people to think about familiar experiences in a new way; for example, 'How would things change for you if you lost some weight?').

The Milan team, Tomm and their followers also highlighted two other central principles: tracking language (picking up and using the exact words that patients use) and following feedback (asking questions based on what the patient has just said rather than the ideas you had in your head).

A MODEL TO UNDERSTAND HOW PATIENTS TELL THEIR STORIES

The narrative medicine movement has been a great philosophical revolution in healthcare. Some of the practical skills and principles I have just described can really help to bring the theoretical and conceptual benefits into the consultation room. But how many doctors or healthcare professionals have any sense of how patients tell their stories? Would you be able to recognise the basic elements of a story, or understand what's missing from an incomplete one? If we are dealing in stories, shouldn't we know what one looks like? There is a model of narratives which I think could be practically helpful for doctors in the consultation.

William Labov, an American sociolinguist who studied hundreds of natural conversations in New York in the 1960s and 1970s (Labov & Waletsky, 1967), concluded that fully formed natural personal narratives have six key ingredients (see Figure 3.2).

While there is debate over the merits and limitations of this model, particularly its focus on events rather than experience (Patterson, 2008), Labov's structural approach has become paradigmatic in the field of personal narrative research – and most investigators either refer to it, use it or adapt it for their own usage (Langellier, 1989). It has been used in researching patients' stories in consultations (Clark & Mishler, 1992) and for our purposes, it seems an evidence-based starting point for making sense of authentic personal narratives – the type that most patients will be telling in consultations.

Here is an explanation of the different elements of Labov's model, along with a few suggestions as to how doctors might make use of it in the consultation.

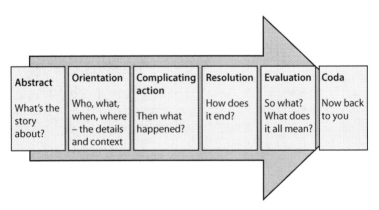

Figure 3.2 Adapted from Labov's sociolinguistic model of personal narratives. (From Labov & Waletsky, 1967.)

ABSTRACT [OPENING]

This is a short summary of what is to come. In medical settings, the abstract might be 'It's my headaches doctor, they've been getting much worse and I don't think I can cope any more ...'. We know that patients often prepare these abstracts at home, or even while waiting in the waiting room – similar to what Neighbour called 'opening gambits' (Neighbour, 2004).

If the abstract is missing or unclear, it is easier for the doctor to ignore or misunderstand the story which follows. The skill here is in choosing an opening invitation that allows the patient to tell their opening in the way they want to. You might use summarising to make sure you have understood, and encourage the patient to tell their whole story, perhaps by active listening, or encouraging noises such as 'Go on ...', or 'Tell me more about that.'

ORIENTATION [DETAILS]

This clause answers the 'Who, What, When and Where' questions. All of us – patients included – can occasionally dwell too much on these details when we are telling our stories: 'It was last Thursday – or was it? No, it was the same day that Anne came round etc. etc.' It may be possible to sensitively 'fast-forward' patients who are stuck on irrelevant details by using phrases such as 'Don't worry too much about the detail at this stage – I'm really keen to hear what happened next.' On the other hand, some detail and characterisation may be vital to create intended meanings and emotions. So beware of hurrying the patient impatiently at this point, as you may miss some important contextual details.

COMPLICATING ACTION [MAIN EVENTS]

This is the core narrative, providing the 'what happened' part of the story. Often in everyday conversation these are simply a sequence of events with some sort of meaning (the basic definition of a narrative). But the classic story is character-driven and has recognisable elements, described neatly by Scholes (1982):

> *a telling or recounting of a string of events with at least three basic elements:*
>
> 1. *a situation involving some predicament, conflict or struggle,*
> 2. *an animate protagonist who engages with this situation for a purpose,*
> 3. *a plot during which the predicament is somehow resolved.*

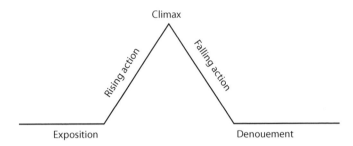

Figure 3.3 Freytag's Pyramid: symbolising his theory of dramatic structure. (Illustration from Wikimedia Commons: http://commons.wikimedia .org/wiki/File:Freytags_pyramid.svg.)

In the classic story, these elements are arranged into a story structure or plot as shown in Figure 3.3.

So how might this be helpful in a consultation? Conflict arises in stories because of some gap or block which is preventing the hero (for us, usually our patient) from achieving their goal. So clarifying the patient's goal or goals, and their motivation, is often key to understanding the patient's story. As doctors, getting to grips with where the conflict is may also be crucial. Conflict may arise from external sources (other people, organisations, illnesses that are seen as 'outside' the person), or from internal sources (self-esteem problems, depression and so on). We need to know where the patient is aiming, and why, and what is preventing them from getting there. Having a stock phrase, such as 'What would be the most helpful thing I could do for you today?' or 'What one thing would help you most?' can be a helpful way to identify and unblock important story conflicts.

RESOLUTION [ENDING, OR DENOUEMENT]

This is the telling of the final key event of a story. Endings aren't always happy, but there needs to be a resolution of some sort. Patients may come to the doctor looking for some resolution to their illness story, and it's the doctor's job to help to find some sort of acceptable resolution with the patient. Sometimes patients will tell a story which already has a resolution – or seems to (for example, 'I had this rash two weeks ago but it's gone now') – and then the doctor must try to understand whether this story needs finishing, what sort of ending the patient was expecting (perhaps it signifies an ongoing illness), or whether it's a different story altogether that needs telling (the story of the patient's allergies for example).

EVALUATION [MEANING]

This section of the model functions to make the point of the story clear; it answers the 'so what?' question. Labov has described evaluation as 'perhaps the most important element in addition to the basic narrative clause' (Labov, 1972) and Riessman calls it the 'soul of the narrative', telling us what the point of the story is, as well as showing us how the narrator wants to be understood (Riessman, 2002). For doctors and patients, this part of the narrative is central to getting at its meaning. It may be expressed as, for example, 'This has never happened to me before – so something serious must be wrong.' But it may not be expressed at all, so your job then is to try to elicit the meaning of the story with the patient. This could translate into finding out their ICE; but there could be a much broader meaning – about values for example.

CODA [HAND-BACK]

This is a signal that the narrative has ended and brings the listener back to the point at which she or he entered the narrative. An example might be: 'Anyway, enough about my day – what about yours?' Or in the consultation: 'So I don't know if you can help me doctor ...' or 'It's probably nothing and I don't want to waste your time, but I thought I'd better come anyway.' It's important that doctors recognise these hand-backs; that's how patients tell us that it's our turn to speak.

Patients' narratives aren't always neat and linear as in the diagram. For example, Labov himself acknowledges that the evaluations – in other words the narrator's explanations about what the story means – are often interspersed throughout the narrative structure, not just at the end. As most doctors are aware, sometimes people start their story halfway through, or at the end. The key is to understand the elements and their purpose in the telling of a personal story.

Some might say that a structural approach like Labov's can lead to a superficial analysis, ignoring the subtleties of human interaction by concentrating too much on what is said rather than how it is said. But a structural approach does not preclude a deeper analysis of how people tell their stories in consultations. Indeed, more in-depth consultation skills such as picking up on cues, and paying attention to body language or paralanguage, may start to make more sense in the context of greater narrative structural understanding.

SUMMARY

The consultation between doctor and patient can be seen as a meeting of stories. A narrative understanding of what goes on during a consultation can offer new insights into the doctor–patient encounter and may encourage a more patient-centred, collaborative approach. There are several practical techniques and principles which can guide practitioners in making the most of this narrative perspective in the consultation, including existing consultation models and skills designed to help patients tell their stories and to co-create a satisfactory shared story. Another potentially helpful tool is the model structure of personal narratives suggested by Labov, which offers practitioners a way to identify and engage with authentic narratives and their key elements.

REFERENCES AND FURTHER READING

Beckman H.B., Frankel R.M. The effect of physician behavior on the collection of data. *Ann. Intern. Med.* 1984; *101*(5): 692–6.

Clark J.A., Mishler E.G. Attending to patients' stories: Reframing the clinical task. *Sociol. Health Illn.* 1992; *14*(3): 344–72.

De Silva D. *Evidence: Helping people share decisions.* London: The Health Foundation; 2012.

Elwyn G., Frosch D., Thomson R., et al. Shared decision making: A model for clinical practice. *J. Gen. Intern. Med.* 2012; *27*(10): 1361–7.

Halpern J. What is clinical empathy? *J. Gen. Intern. Med.* 2003; *18*(8): 670–4.

Hojat M., Louis D.Z., Markham F.W., et al. Physicians' empathy and clinical outcomes for diabetic patients. *Acad. Med.* 2011; *86*(3): 359–64.

Labov W. *Sociolinguistic patterns.* Philadelphia, PA: University of Pennsylvania Press; 1972.

Labov W., Waletsky J. Narrative analysis: Oral versions of personal experience. In: Helms J., ed. *Essays in the verbal and visual arts: Proceedings of the 1966 annual spring meeting of the American Ethnological Society.* Seattle, WA: American Ethnological Society; 1967, pp. 12–44.

Langellier K.M. Personal narratives: Perspectives on theory and research. *Text Perform Q.* 1989; *9*(4): 243–76.

Launer J. *Narrative-based primary care: A practical guide.* Oxford: Radcliffe Medical Press; 2002.

Levinson, W. Physician-patient communication: A key to malpractice prevention. *JAMA.* 1994; *272*(20): 1619–20.

Little P., Everitt E., Williamson I., et al. Observational study of effect of patient centredness and positive approach on outcomes of general practice consultations. *BMJ.* 2001; *323*(7318): 908–11.

Marvel M.K., Epstein R.M., Flowers K., et al. Soliciting the patient's agenda: Have we improved? *JAMA.* 1999; *281*(3): 283–7.

Mercer S.W., Reynolds W.J. Empathy and quality of care. *Br. J. Gen. Pract.* 2002; *52*(Suppl.): S9–12.

Mishler E.G. *The discourse of medicine: Dialectics of medical interviews.* Norwood, NJ: Ablex Publishing; 1984.

Neighbour R. *The inner consultation: How to develop an effective and intuitive consulting style.* 2nd ed. Oxford: Radcliffe Publishing; 2004.

Patterson W. Narratives of events: Labovian narrative analysis and its limitations. In: Andrews M., Squire C., Tamboukou M., eds. *Doing narrative research.* Thousand Oaks, CA: Sage Publications; 2008, p. 176.

Pendleton D., Schofield T., Tate P., et al. *The new consultation: Developing doctor-patient communication.* Oxford: Oxford University Press; 2003.

Riessman C. Narrative analysis. In: Huberman A., Miles M., eds. *The qualitative researcher's companion.* Thousand Oaks, CA: Sage Publications; 2002, pp. 217–70.

Roter D., Hall J. *Doctors talking with patients/patients talking with doctors: Improving communication in medical visits.* 2nd ed. Westport, CT: Praeger; 2006.

Scholes R. *Semiotics and interpretation.* New Haven, CT: Yale University Press; 1982.

Silverman J., Kurtz S., Draper J. *Skills for communicating with patients.* 2nd ed. Oxford: Radcliffe Medical Press; 1998.

Sobel R.J. Eva's stories: Recognizing the poverty of the medical case history. *Acad. Med.* 2000; *75*(1): 85–9.

Stewart M., Brown J.B., Weston W.W., et al. *Patient-centred medicine: transforming the clinical method.* Thousand Oaks, CA: Sage Publications; 1995.

Stewart M., Roter D., eds. *Communicating with medical patients.* Thousand Oaks, CA: Sage Publications; 1989.

THE PATIENT'S STORY, THE DOCTOR'S STORY

Fiona Nicol

We do not see things as they are, we see things as we are.

Anais Nin

In any bookstore, there's a wall of books that patients have written about their illness and a wall of books by doctors writing about their practice; I only wish they would read one another's texts.

Rita Charon

All of us have a story, which has made us who we are today. We carry with us the product of all our experiences, good and bad, and this modifies how we behave in the future. Our lives are built on our personal experience. The same experience affects different people in many different ways and we are all aware of this. How often have you been surprised by the way someone has acted in a particular situation which they have told you about? As a GP, I sometimes felt that I could no longer be surprised by things that people did or said and the way they behaved. However, most days someone would amaze me with their behaviour, at the things they hid from their nearest and dearest and at the consequences these decisions and actions had on their lives and their interactions with others. We need to acknowledge these differences and know about them as doctors and health professionals trying to help others because we are trying to help patients move from one personal space into another where they can see a way forward where previously they were stuck. Our role is: 'to cure sometimes, to relieve often and to comfort always'.

DOI: 10.1201/9781003409151-4

WHY DOES THE PATIENT'S STORY MATTER?

Patients come to us for multiple reasons and many of them are not strictly medical ones. They often present these problems wittingly or unwittingly as physical symptoms as this gives them permission to seek help. We can only fully help them if we have some inkling of what is going on for them, hence the importance of gaining insight into our patient's background stories. If we do so then our interaction is likely to be much more fulfilling and productive for them (and for us). We are seeking to build a partnership with the patient where we have expertise in one area (our theoretical medical knowledge) and the patient in another (their body, mind and back-story). Fully understanding our patients means being less judgemental and condemnatory and enables us to be more empathic. Research has shown that patients are much more likely to listen to what we have to say and follow our advice if they feel understood (Charon, 2008). To be the most effective that we can we have to be genuinely empathic.

BOX 4.1 BACK-STORY

Back-story: A narrative providing a history or background context, especially for a character or situation in a literary work, film or dramatic series. The difference is that with a patient their back-story is not fiction.

A working partnership with patients, even if our meeting lasts only 10 minutes, should leave the patient feeling enabled and better able to deal with their situation. Peter and Elizabeth Tate described how getting to know a patient in general practice is like building a wall (Tate & Tate, 2014). Each time that you see the patient you should build another brick in the wall of your knowledge of that person; this aids your understanding of them and how they deal with life. Over many years in practice you may still not have built a complete wall of knowledge of the patient but you will understand them better. In hospital and as a specialist there is usually much less opportunity to build up this knowledge of the patient. However, you should still use as much information about them, from as many sources as possible, to maximise the effective use of your time together.

The patient's story affects our interaction with them during the consultation, and the consultation is the heart of the therapeutic process. Usually, it is face to face but increasingly it is via phone, email or text. If you are not actually seeing the patient face to face it is even more important to ensure you are fully informed about their story to avoid leaping to inaccurate assumptions about them. Even an apparently simple consultation where someone attends with a cough needs us to fully understand their reasons for attending. They may fear that because this cough has taken longer to go away than normal they have a 'serious' infection requiring antibiotics. If as a child they were taken to the GP with each cough and cold they suffered, and on each occasion the GP prescribed something that apparently effected a cure (as the self-limiting viral infection resolved), they will expect the same thing to happen as an adult. If they have just nursed their father through terminal lung cancer, their anxiety about this as a possible cause is heightened and it is an obvious fear for the GP to seek out and lay bare. These, or other ideas, will be influenced by their past experiences.

HELMAN'S FOLK MODEL

Cecil Helman was a medical anthropologist who also worked for many years as a GP (Helman, 2006). He looked at the cultural factors relating to health and illness and suggested that a patient comes to a doctor seeking answers to six questions.

1. What has happened?
2. Why has it happened?
3. Why to me?
4. Why now?
5. What would happen if nothing were done about it?
6. What should I do about it and whom should I consult for further help?

This is a very task-orientated view of the consultation and makes us focus on the problem through the patient's eyes, not simply through a purely medical model.

To look at a more behavioural style of consulting we can use Eric Berne's model of the human psyche (www.ericberne.com/transactional-analysis). This describes the psyche as existing in one of three states: Parent, Adult or Child. At any given moment each of us is in one of these states of mind and this governs how we think, feel and react. We may be a critical or caring parent, a logical adult or a spontaneous or dependent child. The traditional model of a consultation was that of the parental doctor and the child-like patient. This is not always in the interests of either party. Breaking out of this mould means that we need to recognise what state of mind both we, and the patient, are in. If we are both trying to be parents then our meeting is likely to be dysfunctional and unproductive. For most patients the consultation would ideally be an adult-to-adult interaction.

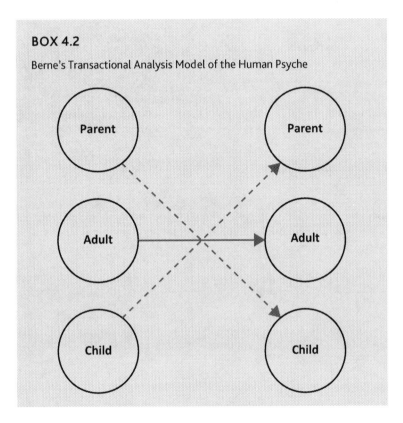

BOX 4.2

Berne's Transactional Analysis Model of the Human Psyche

PAST EXPERIENCE

Patients brought up to regard the doctor as omnipotent may well find it very difficult to engage in a two-way adult process of truly shared care. They have come to believe doctors know best and want the doctor to behave as a caring parent with themselves as the child. These are the patients who ask you which treatment you personally would have if you offer them choices. It can be extremely difficult to disentangle their true ideas about ways forward. It is very easy to slip into simply giving them what you think is best. If the outcome is not beneficial for the patient, they can become stuck and unable to move forward. This leaves you feeling inadequate about how you managed the situation and you may overcompensate by attempting to become a favourable part of the patient's story. Possibly the patient stops seeing you with no word of explanation. Either way the outcome is not ideal for you or the patient. The converse is the doctor who wants to be liked and therefore cannot confront patients about their behaviour. They may allow the patient to act as the critical parent while they are the child. If we are honest with ourselves we may recognise that we want all of our patients to like us. Most of us went into the caring professions because we wanted to help people without any idea that this may entail not always doing as the patient wants or expects. Here, the patient's story may be that they hold a special place in the doctor's affections (and it may be as strong a thought as that) and become dependent on their monthly trip to the health centre. This gives them a story for their friends about the level of their ill-health which is reinforced by the regular need to be seen. Some even try to manipulate the doctor, consciously or subconsciously.

Neighbour describes how two fields of enquiry exist for the doctor and that these may or may not overlap (Neighbour, 2004). There is the need for the clinical information required to make a diagnosis and management plan. Then there is the need for the patient to feel that they have imparted all the information they need to. If you curtail this, it means that they may feel that they have not been adequately attended to. Clinical assessment, although difficult, is seldom a problem; that is what we spend the greater part of our undergraduate career working on. However, all doctors need to develop the ability to elicit the context in which the health problem has arisen and how it now affects the patient. We are all impelled to attribute meaning and significance to events that befall us and which, in turn, affect us. The patient asks themselves: 'Where does this new experience fit into my personal scheme of things?' You should always ask yourself: 'What does this problem mean to this person?' It is this curiosity, combined with the human and cultural heritage that we all share, that will increase the relevance and efficacy of your meetings with patients.

BOX 4.3

Think of the last patient who brought you a gift.

- What was it?
- When did it occur?
- What was the reason they gave it?
- Why to you?
- Why then?
- What might they have wanted from you in exchange?
- What story do you think the patient had told themselves about the interaction between themselves and you when they gave you the gift?
- How did this influence the consultation?

NATURE OR NURTURE?

We are not personally conscious of our birth but we will have heard its story and recognise the inevitable effect on how we are treated by our parents. They experienced our birth uniquely and will remember and react to it, and us, in their own individual way.

The patient's beliefs and motivations will affect whether they accept or reject your advice and suggestions. These are not under your control and, from this, the model of the consultation using ICE developed:

- **I**deas
- **C**oncerns
- **E**xpectations

BOX 4.4

Think of any sets of identical twins that you know.

- Can you tell them apart? How do you do this?
- Are there subtle physical differences?
- Are there mental and emotional differences?
- What has produced these differences, since twins are genetically identical?
- How does each of them see themselves?
- How does this affect how they behave?

The short stories in Box 4.5 illustrate how the manner of our birth, our place in the family and the type of people our parents are will affect us as individuals. Our parents are affected by how they see themselves and their beliefs that are, in turn, affected by their upbringing. Think about your own school days. How did you get on with your peers, younger children, older children? Were your school days happy? Would you go back to your school days or are you deeply glad to have left them behind? What did your teachers think of you and how did they label you? Were you the naughty child, the hard worker, the plodder, the joker, the mischief-maker? We all had labels and either learnt to live with them or spent a long time trying to reject the label and gain a new one, one that accords with our view of ourselves. How successful we were at that then influenced us further.

BOX 4.5

Consider how babies born in the following circumstances may be brought up.

- *How will they think about themselves?*
- *Who will they see themselves as?*
- *What will they tell themselves they are?*

- John and Sophie, age 36 and 37, both professionals, married for 10 years and trying to conceive for five years before paying for IVF. After three unsuccessful cycles Sophie is delighted when she becomes pregnant. Hypertension and occasional vaginal bleeding complicate the pregnancy. She delivers a preterm baby at 30 weeks. The baby is in the special care baby unit for four weeks before being allowed home and is bottle-fed in spite of Sophie struggling to establish breastfeeding.
- Crystalle is 16. She lives at home with her mother who is a single parent living on benefits. She has no siblings and feels ignored by her mother and does not see any other family members. She has had several boyfriends who have used her more as a 'trophy' than as a companion or friend. She gets pregnant by one of them but is not sure which one. She keeps the baby as she 'wants somebody to love'. Her pregnancy is uneventful despite infrequent attendance at antenatal clinics. She has a normal delivery at term and the baby is a good weight. They are discharged with bottle-feeding well established.
- Chris and Jane are in their mid-30s and unmarried. They have known each other since they were 16 and have four children aged three to nine. Chris works in a call centre as a manager and they live near both their parents. Jane is a homemaker looking after the family but is also a child-minder for two other children at the local primary school. She sees herself as an 'earth mother' and many of the local children love going to her house to play and eat her baking. The midwife delivers her fifth child at home with no complications. Breastfeeding is quickly established and the baby thrives in the kitchen, the hub of the busy family life.

Who were our friends? Did we seek them out because we had already decided the type of person we wanted to be and so associated with the same type or did we get on with other like-minded individuals without realising it? Were we very sociable and made lots of friends and belonged to a large circle of friends or were we insular and loners who did not apparently need anyone else?

Were we first to be picked for the general knowledge quiz and last for the football team or vice versa? Was what we told ourselves about ourselves really true? Did we hide from ourselves the fact that we found it very difficult to make friends and would have given anything to be part of a circle of people? How did we cope with the many complex feelings engendered by this situation? Were we picked on and bullied or even abused?

BOX 4.6

Sandra was one of two children born in the 1960s to a middle-class couple. James, her brother, was five years younger. Her father was a manager in a local factory and her mother a secretary working part-time in the local solicitor's office. At primary school, Sandra was always in the top five of the class and learnt to read and write and fit in with her peer group with no difficulty. She was gregarious and popular with her classmates. James started at the same school with the same teacher who had initially taught Sandra. One day he heard the teacher talking to his mother as she was picking him up saying, 'What a shame he is not as clever as Sandra.' Already he felt in some way he had failed, and he was only five! His parents sought some expert help to see why he was not learning to read and write as quickly as Sandra and he was diagnosed as being dyslexic. The experts decided that James was really left-handed and he was retaught to hold his pen in his left hand. All this took over one year, a sixth of his life so far.

- Think about how this formative experience could have moulded James's long-term perceptions about himself.
- How might it have influenced his relationship with the teacher and parents both then and in the future?
- If you think that he was too young to really take much notice of these comments, consider whether this might always be true.
- How might James's beliefs about himself have influenced who he became and how he coped with adversity, including illness, as an adult?

How did we relate to our parents? Did we feel truly loved and accepted totally for who we were or did we feel overt or subtle pressure to conform to an ideal that our parents had for us? Can we, even now as mature adults, think back honestly about our relationship with them? Did we reject their ideas for us or did we embrace them knowing we were subverting ourselves to their wishes and vicarious ideas? What about our siblings? Who did they think they were and how did they see themselves in the family? How did that affect our relationship with them and within the family unit?

Our upbringing and past life experiences affect the way we behave, particularly when we become ill or believe ourselves to be ill. If you are used to using your brain and have many opportunities to think and interact with others during a day, you may wonder how people who work on a production line feel about the day and how they get through it without the mental stimulation that you have. Do they see themselves as a part of the machine that produces the final object they are manufacturing or is it simply a means to an end? All these events lodge themselves in the subconscious mind and are part of the person's 'back-story'. People believe many things that are manifestly untrue. However, whether true or not, honestly and mistakenly believing something is true will still affect the person concerned. They may see themselves as a failure, someone to whom 'bad things' happen and that these events are decreed by fate and not under their control. Others may see themselves as very powerful and in total command of their fate. Some people believe they are watched over by a guardian angel that looks after them even when things go wrong. It is not difficult to see how any of these extreme positions will affect how a person reacts to a serious illness. All of us have a character and personality shaped by events in our back-story. We tell ourselves things about what happens to us and this, in turn, affects our mood and the outcome of events.

BOX 4.7

Think of your last consultation that went really well or really badly.

- How would you describe the patient?
- How would the patient describe you?
- Think of five adjectives to describe yourself and the patient.
- What makes these true?

These terms may vary according to the time that you are thinking about yourself or the situation in which you interviewed this patient. Which would you use to describe your long-term character and personality? Would colleagues agree with you; if not how would others describe you?

Some people accept blame. They tell themselves that they will never be successful, but we need to understand how they define success. Their ideas may be grandiose and unrealistic so they set themselves up to fail and therefore the story about being unsuccessful is perpetuated. Others may tell themselves they are bound to succeed and yet their goals are modest. They may build on this success to set higher and higher goals, always managing to achieve them. Some manage to rise above their problems while others sink beneath the waves of everyday problems.

BOX 4.8

Work with a colleague. Think of a patient whom you have both seen professionally. Independently write down five phrases to describe them. Compare notes.

- What terms are the same and which are different?
- What does each of you bring to the interaction with that particular individual that leads you to describe them in these terms?
- Imagine how the patient might describe themselves and write those words down.
- How does this differ from your and your colleague's descriptions?
- Why might these words be different?
- What does the patient know about themselves that you do not?

Often our descriptions of patients seem judgemental rather than understanding.

These previous experiences affect anyone facing their own mortality. If they develop an inoperable cancer or progressive debilitating neurological condition like Parkinson's disease, their past experience will affect how they meet the challenge and how they react when things do not go as they hope and plan. Our understanding of why some people seem totally accepting when things go wrong and others are incensed by small things going wrong will enable us to be more empathic and effective clinicians.

BOX 4.9

Think of expressions you have heard colleagues use about patients and write them down. (Examples might include old, crumbly, chatty, nervous, demanding, rude, angry, beautiful, huge, boring, tedious, mad, smelly, barking, arrogant etc., etc.)

- Consider why the patients might have seemed like their description.
- Summarise what the real underlying person may have been feeling underneath your one-word description.
- How might this have been influenced by their past experiences?

HOW DOES THE DOCTOR FIT INTO THE PATIENT'S STORY?

We do not get up in the morning and go to work setting out to upset people. Yet listening to some stories that people tell about their experiences with doctors or other health professionals, you could believe that was the case. There is sometimes a huge rift between what we set out to do and the actual outcome. We can have a benign or a malign influence on the patient that sits with us in the consultation. We all aim to be beneficent and not to make our patient's situation worse. We do not want to become part of the patient's story about not being heard or listened to or dismissed or pushed into undertaking treatment that was at best unhelpful and at worst positively dangerous.

BEARING WITNESS

Iona Heath talks about how doctors bear witness to a patient's suffering (Heath, 2008). We may not be able to do much and indeed should become adept at not interfering where we may make the situation worse by over-medicalising a problem or adding medication to no benefit. We should never overlook the importance of actively listening to a patient's story and simply acknowledging what has happened to them. To do this we have to develop what Rita Charon calls 'narrative competence'. She defines this as the ability to acknowledge, absorb, interpret and act on the stories and the plights of others. She suggests that we actively learn to do this. Many doctors already do this unconsciously, but we can become more aware and practised in the technique by learning to closely read literature and adopting reflective writing. Charon hypothesises that this allows practitioners to reach out and join their patients in illness and help to bridge the divide between physicians and patients and colleagues. She believes that this offers fresh opportunities for respectful, nourishing and empathic medical care. Her work has produced a field called narrative medicine – the act of becoming more adept at listening to and hearing patients' stories.

NARRATIVE COMPETENCE

Narrative knowledge is how we understand and make sense of the meaning and significance of stories that patients tell us. This provides us with a deeper, richer and more effective understanding of their situation and contrasts sharply with our 'medical' understanding of a person. Medical knowledge is essential but is dispassionately scientific and is applied across the board to many different situations and people. So, for example, we know the symptoms and signs of acute appendicitis but we have to use this factual knowledge within the context of the individual sitting with us complaining of abdominal pain. Doing this within the context of the patient's story allows us to make more accurate judgements about the likelihood of this pain requiring surgery. Alternatively, by sitting, listening and bearing witness to their current life situation in which they feel trapped and which has caused a flare-up in their irritable bowel syndrome the outcome may be much improved for the patient.

Telling a story requires a listener; it is a two-way process and so we should not be surprised when patients feel deeply unhappy if they feel that they have not been heard. Many complaints about doctors stem from an initial communication failure from which the relationship between the doctor and patient never fully recovers. True engagement transforms both of us forever. The change may be small and subtle but it is present. Once fully engaged with the patient's story we can much better understand their experiences.

Psychoanalysts understand that the act of narrating their story is a central therapeutic act for the patient. They suggest that this is because finding the words to describe the disorder and the worries generated by it gives a shape to it and some degree of control over the chaos caused by the illness. As we listen we can imagine the effects each situation has had on the narrator. What we often neglect is our need to imagine the biological and the social consequences: how this has affected them, their family, friends and colleagues. Similarly, we need to understand the patient's cultural background and its effect on their day-to-day life.

True empathy has consequences for the doctor and produces a dilemma. As doctors we try to avoid becoming too attached to patients to allow us to provide an objective view, yet true empathy demands emotional resonance. We must be aware of this dichotomy (Halpern, 2003).

HOW MAY WE DEVELOP NARRATIVE COMPETENCE?

Charon teaches that to become competent at analysing narrative you should assess a written story in five ways (Box 4.10).

BOX 4.10

One system to analyse stories (after Charon):

- Frame
- Form
- Time
- Plot
- Desire

Frame: This is the scope of the story and the author's intent. In medicine the frame is often drawn so tightly that we miss vitally important observations because our interest is restricted to the biological. We need to expand our frame of reference and consider all parts of the patient's story.

Form: This encompasses six parts.

- *Genre*: Genre is the type of story, e.g., is it didactic, an epic, a tragedy, a comedy, an allegory or satire?
- *Visible structure*: Does the story have one or is it chaotic?
- *Narrator*: From whose point of view is the story told?
- *Metaphors*: Some anthropologists think that all life is a metaphor as that is how the human brain works. Does the story have obvious metaphors or is it one big metaphor that can tell us more about how the teller sees things?
- *Diction*: Is the style and tone of voice adopted in the story? Is it abstruse and scholarly or emotional and seeking to influence and persuade? Is it colloquial and easy to understand with less apparent depth?
- *Time*: What period does the story cover? Is it told chronologically or does it jump around? Does the order of telling the events indicate their relative importance?

Plot: What events make up the story? Do they relate to one another in a pattern, in a sequence, through cause and effect, how the reader views the story or simply by coincidence?

Desire: What appetite was satisfied by reading the story and what is satisfied for the teller or writer? Think about whether any desires are awoken in you by reading or hearing the story. If you can more clearly identify your needs and longings and what the story has accomplished this may echo those of the writer or storyteller.

Of course, there is a considerable difference between closely analysing a written text and sitting listening to a patient's story. However, by honing our critical faculties we can become more open to the patient's story by learning to actively listen. We actively listen by delving into our own memory and associations and using our creative powers and experience from others to identify meaning. Sometimes this is just not possible, as the narrator's story is so outwith our experience that we cannot connect or make sense of what we are told. Then, our role is simply to act as an empathic listener bearing witness to a patient's suffering.

A problem that affects all health practitioners is lack of time. This may be particularly difficult if we only see the patient on one occasion. Lack of continuity of care in primary care, with the patient seeing many different doctors with the same problem, may aggravate the problem. Not unreasonably, people become exhausted telling their story multiple times, going over the same ground with little progress. This is particularly a concern in hospital where the patient may have to repeat the same story to an Emergency Department receptionist, triage nurse, junior doctor, radiographer, specialist and so on.

We have to find more powerful methods of developing the therapeutic relationship. Charon contends that learning narrative skills can counter this pressure. Once we learn to affirm people's strength, accept their weaknesses, become familiar with suffering even if we do not experience it ourselves and be able to truly understand individuals then we become more able to utilise effectively a hugely powerful tool in our armamentarium. This tool is ourselves – 'the Doctor'. Balint first described the power of the drug 'Doctor' and by developing our narrative skills we can develop into more effective users of our own personality and abilities (Balint, 1964).

BOX 4.11 A PATIENT'S STORY

Annette was a 40-year-old single mother I saw regularly. She worked hard in two part-time cleaning jobs. Her husband had left her with two children under five yet everything she did was to try to support them and allow them to grow up to be independent adults. She had the most poorly controlled asthma I had ever seen. Her jobs did not help as she was clearly allergic to house dust. She had been on depot steroid injections for several years. She and I agreed to try to wean her off them and control her asthma using inhalers with oral steroids for acute attacks. Every time we tried to reduce her steroids her asthma got worse. We tried everything including hospital admission, oral steroid-sparing agents, even homeopathy. Nothing worked. Indeed her symptoms were probably best when she was admitted for a week to the homeopathic hospital. On reflection, this was a time when she had no responsibilities and felt nurtured and cared for.

I noticed that emotional distress coincided with deterioration in her asthma. In any other person this would simply have meant increasing inhaled steroids and regular use of bronchodilators, but since I was responsible for changing the dose of her injected steroids to cope with the exacerbations I was all too aware of the physical changes wrought by her emotional problems. Year in, year out, she coped with the increasing side effects of her more labile asthma and high-dose systemic steroids. She developed the full litany of side effects: early cataracts, central obesity, hypertension, osteoporotic fracture, peripheral vascular disease and Type 2 diabetes. After many years she was nearly housebound. After another injection and discussion about steroid reduction, she suddenly turned to me at the door and said: 'I would like to contact my daughter.' I had thought I knew all about her story but this was the first I had heard of a daughter. 'I never told you about her. I was scared to. I haven't told anyone about her,' she said.

Clearly, I had not listened attentively enough. It had taken her years to find the courage to tell me her secret. I asked her back in to the consulting room. Out tumbled the heart-rending story of her becoming pregnant at 16 at a time when this was completely unacceptable in society. She was still living at home with her parents as her pregnancy advanced. She delivered the baby in a convent in the countryside not far from where she lived. She had just over 24 hours with the baby and then her mother and father came to visit. Her mother sat by the bed while her father picked up the baby and took it outside into the corridor. When he returned a few minutes later he no longer held the baby. He told her that she would never see the baby again and she never had from that day onwards.

Why did she suddenly feel able to tell me after all those years? 'Because I couldn't keep it in any longer and you knew everything else about me,' she told me.

What emotional effect must this event have had on a young girl in her situation? I now understood why any emotional stress might trigger her asthma. I could change nothing but I could bear witness to her suffering then and now.

BOX 4.12

Stanley was mandated on to my list of patients. He was 55, unemployed and on benefits. Previous GPs had been unable to cope with his demanding, unpredictable behaviour. Our first meeting went reasonably well. I agreed to find out from his previous GP what painkillers he was taking and see him the following day. It was clear that he was addicted to prescribed analgesics but he still suffered continual pain in his head and neck. This pervaded him, affecting his ability to do anything during the day and stopping him from sleeping at night. Over the next weeks he told me his story: He never knew his parents and had been brought up in an orphanage. He became a pipefitter in the local docks but many years previously he had been blown up when his oxyacetylene torch ignited explosive gases in a pipe he was working on. The pipe had landed across his neck. Since then he had been in pain which he was adamant was not helped by anything.

The pain affected Stanley's whole demeanour. He constantly screwed his eyes up and moved his shoulders around within his outsized coat to try to find some relief. He found it very difficult to engage in eye contact or sit still. Over the following months I attempted all the usual well-documented ways of helping him to control the number of drugs he took, but without success. He remained dependent on them and constantly tried to increase the dose to stop the pain. He kept looking for a miracle cure to take away the pain forever.

One day he came to see me and thrust a scrap of paper at me. It was a page torn from a child's exercise book. On it were several rectangles in two rows bordered by a box. One rectangle was shaded in. Stanley explained to me that the shaded box was the position of his bed in the orphanage. He had drawn a plan diagram of the room he lived in and exactly where his bed was in relation to the door and the window. He had slept there from the age of five till he was 16 and turned out of the orphanage. He had nowhere to go, no family, no job, no training. He hated the orphanage's staff. I asked why since they had provided him with food, clothing and shelter. He told me about the punishments for misdemeanours. This had included standing on a chair in the corner of the room with the 12 beds in it and a board round his neck with 'Dunce' written on it. This had been administered regularly for minor misdemeanours. He had felt totally humiliated. As he spoke, he wept.

It was hard to imagine the effect this had, although I could see the end result before me. 'No one ever let me tell them about it before,' he said, before he took back the scrap of paper, turned and left the consulting room. I could not change what had happened but I could simply listen to his story. At least I now understood the impossibility of ever trying to stop his pain.

He still came to see me regularly. He managed to limit his intake of medication, although he always remained dependent.

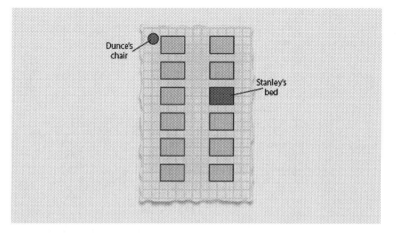

BOX 4.13

The patient's story is important because of the following.

- It provides meaning, context and perspective of the patient's situation.
- It defines the
    - WHY
    - HOW
    - IN WHAT WAY
    - They are ill.
- Understanding it allows us to help the patient reframe the story in another way that makes sense to them.
- If we hear it effectively, it encourages empathy and promotes understanding between the patient and us.
- It may offer clues about the underlying diagnosis.
- Hearing it encourages a holistic approach to the patient.
- Telling it is intrinsically therapeutic.

STORIES THAT PATIENTS TELL THEMSELVES ABOUT THEIR SEEING THE DOCTOR

Think about the last patient you saw where you felt things had not gone as well as they might have. What had the patient told themselves about the trip to see you before the consultation? How did the patient regard themselves?

What story had they told themselves about the consultation they were going to have with you? This depends largely on their past experience with doctors but also their expectations if they have met you before.

For instance, if they have previously had an X-ray for low back pain, your suggestion that there may be a different and better way forward is likely to be met with disbelief. Your attempts to involve them in an adult-to-adult discussion about the way forward may be met with resistance. They seek to deal with you as a child, telling you what they want and digging their heels in.

BOX 4.14 EXAMPLES

- A young woman struggling to cope in an urban flat with two young children; she feels she has a right to expect the state or other people to help her.
- An older man in a very senior position in a profession who has had to take time out of his self-imposed busy schedule to get something that he wants from a much younger professional (you – the doctor). He sees himself as very important, exceptionally busy, indispensable and used to having everything go his own way.

Someone worried they have cancer may well expect a referral to a specialist. This story may take some time for a GP to change to a more appropriate one, but first you have to understand the patient's story, why they are sitting with you and what their expectations are.

How often have you been amazed and disappointed by how doctors and health professionals are portrayed on TV or in films? These frequently stereotypical portrayals colour many people's ideas about how doctors behave and set their expectations. Only through their own personal experience will this change and it may take some time to achieve. We try to avoid a situation where they are so disappointed that they vote with their feet and do not return. People do end up seeing the GP that they feel most comfortable with and you should not be disappointed in yourself if that doctor is not you. However much we try to be all things to all our patients it is not always possible. One of the benefits of working in a group or team is that patients have a choice about whom they see.

CONCLUSIONS

Every story requires a narrator and a listener. The story process allows a health practitioner to better understand the patient and the act of telling the story is itself therapeutic. It allows us to bear witness to a patient's suffering even if we cannot alleviate it directly. Each story is unique to that individual. The same story told by another person will be different but no less true.

Stories allow us to learn more about ourselves and to consider and learn about other areas such as ethics. When we listen we have to decide if the teller is reliable or not. We need to consider what the story is really about. Is it a metaphor for some other distress or happening? What or whose angle is it told from? Whose voice is being heard and why? What type of language is being used?

Stories may tend to overlap and need to be drawn together. The story of illness has many different interpretations. Ultimately the patient is the author of their own truth but, as you listen, you can support them to reframe it. Together you can help it make more sense to them and enable them to take more control over the direction. By truly hearing and empathising with the patient you will become a more effective doctor.

REFERENCES AND FURTHER READING

Balint M. *The doctor, his patient and the illness*. 2nd ed. Edinburgh: Churchill Livingstone; 1964, reprinted 1986.

Charon R. *Narrative medicine: Honoring the stories of illness*. New York: Oxford University Press; 2008.

Halpern J. What is clinical empathy? *J. Gen. Intern. Med.* 2003; *18*: 670–4.

Heath I. *Matters of life and death: Key writings*. Oxford: Radcliffe Publishing; 2008.

Helman C.G. *Suburban Shaman: Tales from medicine's front line*. London: Hammersmith Press; 2006.

Neighbour R. *The inner consultation: How to develop an effective and intuitive consulting style*. 2nd ed. Oxford: Radcliffe Publishing; 2004.

Tate P., Tate E. *The doctor's communication handbook*. 7th ed. London: Radcliffe Publishing; 2014.

CHILDREN AND STORY

Jim Huntley

Mankind owes to the child the best it has to give.

Geneva Declaration of the Rights of the Child, 1924

I don't know whether you have ever seen a map of a person's mind. Doctors sometimes draw maps of other parts of you, and your own map can become intensely interesting, but catch them trying to draw a map of a child's mind, which is not only confused, but keeps going round all the time. There are zigzag lines on it, just like your temperature on a card, and these are probably roads in the island, for the Neverland is always more or less an island, with astonishing splashes of colour here and there, and coral reefs and rakish-looking craft in the offing, and savages and lonely lairs, and gnomes who are mostly tailors, and caves through which a river runs, and princes with six elder brothers, and a hut fast going to decay, and one very small old lady with a hooked nose. It would be an easy map if that were all, but there is also first day at school, religion, fathers, the round pond, needlework, murders, hangings, verbs that take the dative, chocolate pudding day, getting into braces, say ninety-nine, three-pence for pulling out your tooth yourself, and so on, and either these are part of the island or they are another map showing through, and it is all rather confusing, especially as nothing will stand still.

Of course the Neverlands vary a good deal. John's, for instance, had a lagoon with flamingos flying over it at which John was shooting, while Michael, who was very small, had a flamingo with lagoons flying over it. John lived in a boat turned upside down on the sands, Michael in a wigwam, Wendy in a house of leaves deftly sewn together. John had no friends, Michael had friends at night, Wendy had a pet wolf forsaken by its parents, but on the whole the Neverlands have a family resemblance,

DOI: 10.1201/9781003409151-5

and if they stood still in a row you could say of them that they have each other's nose, and so forth. On these magic shores children at play are for ever beaching their coracles. We too have been there; we can still hear the sound of the surf, though we shall land no more.

(From J M Barrie, 'Peter breaks through',
Chapter 1 in: *Peter and Wendy*, 1911)

My children already recognise me as a false prophet: I serially predict accidents which fail to transpire. They are unimpressed by my argument that pre-emptive action in the light of anticipatable consequences can mitigate against subsequent catastrophe. I explain that accidents and mistakes (apart from neutral or serendipitously advantageous genetic mutations) are best avoided, and you can go a long way to tilt the odds in your favour. They yawn. They have heard it all before and, with every non-occurrence, my credibility falls. As my stock decreases, so does the probability of influence. How often can a parent cry wolf?

We are in the car, negotiating the congested one-way High Street of a coastal town. The sun slants across the red-brick buildings, the pavement and the road. There are swathes of light and shadow; everyone has come out to play. The pavements are narrow, too narrow for two abreast, so people, especially children, dance briefly in the road, springing a quickstep in and out of the traffic. Seemingly every child has an ice cream, except for the smiling four year old bouncing the ball.

I explain to my children that bouncing a football by the roadside is 'crazy'. I say 'crazy' rather than 'stupid', but I mean 'stupid', not that the child is stupid, nor the parent. The bouncing football will miscue, and spring outwards into the road. In the next instant, the boy will see the ball at its zenith, and, scrabbling, reach out after it, leaning into the road. It will happen so fast, before he's thought about what he's doing; he will reach after his ball; he will dive into the path of man's invention. From there it is just luck: how tight are the vehicles, how slow is the car, how close is the car, how alert is the driver, how good are the brakes?

Bouncing a ball by the roadside. *Please* don't do it. I think my children resent my perspective on risk. A skewed perspective, my wife tells me. It is a beautiful sunny day. Everyone is happy. A child is bouncing a ball. I am the only person worried: alone with the black swan event, the prospects of childhood accident, that one particular Borgesian branching path (Borges, 1970).

Maybe we need to discover some things for ourselves. We learn better from mistakes than anticipation. 'Real life' teaches us the harshest lessons, and we 'grow up'. Or do we? It is hard to make the case once you have seen the alcohol-fuelled carnage of a UK adult

Emergency Department on a Friday night. At least when children hurt themselves, they have generally been doing something sensible like skateboarding, climbing a tree or using a trampoline.

In our little enclave of seven houses, our garden is the only one deprived of a trampoline. I have explained laboriously, repeatedly, how people injure themselves on a PFG ('Paediatric Fracture Generator'). They miss the edge, land on their head and break their neck. When multiple people bounce at the same time, it's out of control, people go too high, too wayward, they land on the edge or awkwardly on someone else, breaking almost anything (see Figure 5.1a,b). When the trampoline is on a slope, it is asking for trouble. Safety nets might be helpful, but they can trip you up. Trick moves are dangerous. There is no place for this 'toy of Satan' in my garden. Of course, my children just go next door.

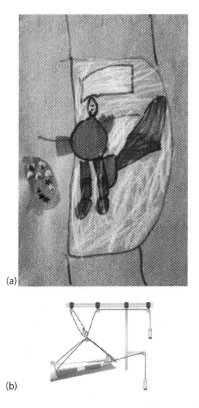

(a)

(b)

Figure 5.1 (a) Self-portrait by five-year-old girl with femoral fracture in Thomas splint (fixed skin traction and balanced suspension); (b) Textbook diagram (Huntley, 2013): my alternative perspective.

When George Nissen and Larry Griswold built the first one in 1936 (McDermott et al., 2006), they could hardly have foreseen the fun. The following year, they added an 'e' to the Spanish word for 'diving-board' and registered 'Trampoline' as a trademark. It is ironic that the two inventors came from the University of Iowa, an institution that has made outstanding world-leading contributions to children's ortho-paedics and trauma (Kavanagh et al., 2013): treatment of club foot, hip dysplasia (abnormal development) and scoliosis.

To be fair, George and Larry did not anticipate that the trampoline would cause childhood injuries on a billion-dollar scale (McDermott et al., 2006). In 2008, a group analysed all forearm fractures presenting to a Glasgow hospital (Bell et al., 2012): 7% were due to trampolines. It's difficult to say if this is too many. If it was 1%, I'd shrug it off. If 25%, I'd lead the campaign to ban them.

In my clinic, children always ask when they can go back to football; it's nearly always football – it looms high in their consciousness (Figure 5.2). In the south of Scotland, sport accounts for 30% of adult tibial frac-tures, and football accounts for just over 80% of these (Court-Brown & McBirnie, 1995). No one is seriously calling for a ban on football. Or should they? In the UK, no back garden landscape is complete without a trampoline. Trampolines and football – they are just facts of life.

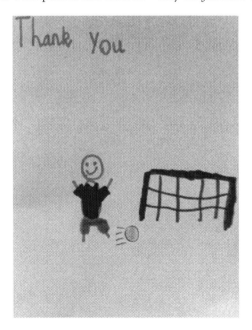

Figure 5.2 Boy and football. Thank-you note from four-year-old boy, on cast removal, keen to return to sport.

Children. How can I introduce this teeming cast of thousands on thousands, so varied? They are migrants cast up on the shore, across history and continents, through all the vagaries of chance and fortune: satires of circumstance. Here are confidence and doubt, affluence and destitution, security, a smile, humour (Figure 5.3), suffering, balloons, kites, footballs, rashes and simple watchfulness: the barometer of despair. Here again, those two imposters (Kipling, 1910): triumph and disaster.

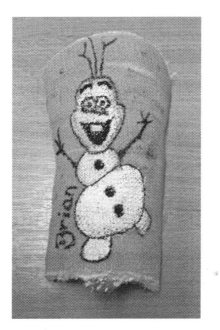

Figure 5.3 Cast art/humour.

Geography recapitulates history, whether through ignorance, or circumstances of science, politics, sociology, economy or culture. One hundred and fifty years ago in the UK, child mortality (0–5 years) was 25%. It declined markedly over the subsequent century (Figure 5.4; Rosling & Zhang, 2011; Rosling, 2013). Similar traces are given for Ethiopia, Australia and the United States. The problem and causes of child mortality were well understood – in 1860, a Glasgow doctor listed in order of importance the five main causes of infantile death (Robertson, 1972):

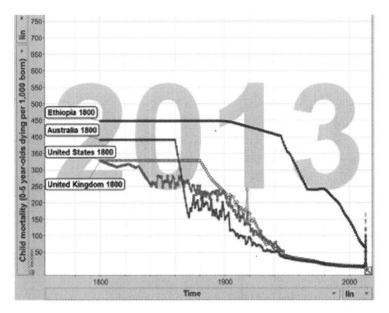

Figure 5.4 Child mortality (0–5 years), as number per 100 live births, by country, 1800–2015. (From www.gapminder.org.)

- Overcrowding and vitiated air, together with poor drainage and inadequate light
- Deficient nutrition
- Want of a hospital for sick children
- Early marriages
- Neglect of illegitimate children

Dr Russell, the medical officer for health in Glasgow in the 1880s, went to the poorest areas of the city, documenting first-hand the deprivation and proportionately grim mortality (Robertson, 1972):

> *There they die, and their little bodies are laid on a table or on a dresser, so as to be somewhat out of the way ... From beginning to rapid ending the lives of these children are short parts in a continuous tragedy.*

Given the recognition of the true nature of the problem – and its solution – the question concerning child mortality is: Should (or could) the pace of change have been quicker? If we take our time increment (the period over which we might make meaningful change) to be a year, the pace of change seems slow. An index, like mortality, is a unitary outcome contingent on an array of variables, many with cultural determinants that are themselves time-heavy (building and staffing a hospital; designing and building a sewerage system; changing a culture to mandate the education of women and children). Other factors involve the uptake of innovations in practice which may require a long period before being accepted and adopted (Rogers, 2003). It may be more appropriate for the time increment to be a human generation, approximately 25 years (Matthews & Hamilton, 2009). If this were the case, then we would ascribe only seven comparator values to our x-axis. Maybe we've done okay. It depends, how you spin it.

In the privileged enclave of the UK, the focus has shifted away from mortality, away from children 'born to die', to children 'born to fail'. Wedge and Prosser encapsulated this shift in their concise, photographically unflinching analysis of the implications of social disadvantage (Wedge & Prosser, 1973). They looked at family composition, number of children/number of parents, low income and poor housing, and showed that 'the disadvantaged group' had 'substantially diminished prospects of normal development' from the very day and circumstances of their births. They concluded with two critical questions:

- As a society, do we really care sufficiently about our children to reduce drastically the hardships of their families?
- Do we care that so many are born to fail?

In 2013, Richard Horton, editor of the *Lancet*, described a short film depicting an infant's response when its mother's interaction was blunted to stillness; there was progressive and escalating distress followed by withdrawal. This is a version of the 'still-face paradigm', an experiment developed by Tronick and colleagues (Brazelton et al., 1975; Tronick et al., 1978; Mesman et al., 2009). Tronick's film (2015) makes awkward viewing: the message is that early social interaction, attachment and relationship are fundamental for healthy child development. Increasingly it is recognised that there are 'serve and return' interactions in early life between child and caregiver, and that these are critical to the development of intricate brain architecture. In terms of human potential, we reap what we sow. Neglect is the most prevalent form of child maltreatment; children who experience it have a greater likelihood of deficits in cognition, executive functions and attention regulation (Center on the Developing Child, 2012, 2015).

The BBC documentary *Child of Our Time* sought to popularise child development (Livingstone, 2008). Lord Winston was the 'face' of the series (Winston, 2006). It is noteworthy that he focused on well-being and happiness rather than achievement per se (Winston, 2006; Livingstone, 2008):

> *Happiness ... has become the holy grail of Modern Society. But adult happiness is largely determined by what happened to us as children ... We must be careful about our aspirations for children. Happiness, content-ment and wisdom are not achieved by fame, and that's a real issue for our society.*

Winston also cautions against value judgements concerning our perceptions of the environment in which a child is brought up. He emphasises the importance of love and support, rather than tidiness and cleanliness per se (Rabinovitch, 2004). He gives his impression of the series, referring to the title of the documentary, when he observes that child education/nurturing/development is an intrinsic reciprocal of society at large (Taylor-Whiffen, 2005):

> *It's like a mirror ... the epithet* Child of Our Time *... is proving very appropriate. It's an archive of the way our society looks at itself ...* Child of Our Time *is not just about the child, it's about* our *time.*

Dr Livingstone, responsible for the series, emphasised the contribution of play and laughter (Livingstone, 2008):

> *Our most surprising findings were about play. Play is vital; it is what makes children happy, as we discovered when we counted the number of laughs. The more children play, the more they laugh, especially when they are outside.*

Later, she quotes the psychologist Professor Belsky (Livingstone, 2008):

> *We've lost sight of the fact that one can have fun and not worry about future consequences but stay in the moment. We don't value the moment, especially in childhood.*

The gap between potential and achievement persists. There is the danger of a fundamental intergenerational failure. As parents, elders, doctors, species ... how are we doing? Who keeps the score and writes our report? What would our report card say? And there are report cards – for dimensions of comparative child well-being in richer countries (UNICEF, 2007, 2011). They make very uncomfortable reading for both the UK and the US.

THE CROCODILE IS TICKING

More recently, Horton commented on the ethics (or otherwise) of global health objectives (Horton, 2015). He used a version of Singer's drowning-child thought experiment (Singer, 1972, 1997) to introduce the concept that ethical obligation is no longer dependent on geography (because of developments in transport technology) or on the actions of others. Singer asks his students to imagine that on their way to class on campus, they pass a shallow pond in which a child seems to be drowning. Rescuing the child would be easy enough but would entail getting wet and dirty, and being late for class. The first question is: 'Do you have an obligation to rescue the child?' By common assent, it seems that the merit of saving the child far outweighs the inconvenience cost. Singer continues:

> *Does it make a difference that there are other people walking past the pond who would equally be able to rescue the child but are not doing so?*

The chorus to the negative is taken to mean that the inaction of others does not justify inaction on our own part.

If we combine Horton's two concerns, the one of child development, the other of universal responsibility, then worldwide perhaps we have an obligation to nurture and sustain our children through to their potential.

One problem is that not everyone wants to fulfil their 'potential'. Back in that UK Emergency Department, I am struck by the volume of *H. 'sapiens'* intent on self-destruction, those falling short by some way of their potential. A partially related concern is the definition of 'potential'. Or, rather, its subject matter and context: the potential for what and on whose authority and within which culture and within what environment?

In two eloquent letters, 20 years apart, Dr Eunson highlights the importance of aid priorities being determined locally rather than imposed by the 'developed' world:

> *We do not need slogans, because it is part of our inheritance to know our problems. We will develop ourselves, so that our progress is part of ourselves.*
>
> *To impose development on a nation, however well-meaning, is a form of colonialism that has burdened the world for too long.*
>
> (Eunson, 1984)

In his second correspondence (Eunson, 2004), he describes a village being asked by a benevolent aid organisation for its key development priorities. It was presumed that the answer would be 'a health centre, school, or irrigation system'. When the reply was 'a football pitch' (football again), the organisation retracted its offer. In Eunson's words:

> *The villagers built their own football pitch, and this engendered such a feeling of community spirit that they built their own health centre the next year without outside help.*

In the harshest of environments, and back with mortality (rather than, necessarily, 'potential'), a consequentialist standpoint mandates saving those who can support others, so that ultimately the greatest good is done by the greatest number. The daily cannula, if there is only one, goes to the otherwise healthy young man who will subsequently feed and support his young family. Albeit with anguish, this affirms rather than negates the maxim from the Geneva Declaration of the Rights of the Child:

> *Mankind owes to the child the best it has to give.*

I believe that human nature – as well as experience and education – is a stratal phenomenon: its nature is initially liquid, like geological silt, and it takes much of its form from the underlying template. Possibly, we can improve ourselves, just as pupils' comprehension is built on that of their teachers, the pioneers of the generation before. In Sir Isaac Newton's words:

> *If I have seen further it is by standing on the shoulders of Giants.*

Schaffer discusses the development of human psychology in such terms (Schaffer, 2004):

> *Human nature cannot be described in the abstract; whatever course children's mental growth takes is to a large extent a function of the cultural tools that are handed down to them by other people.*

Half a century ago, the Goertzels concluded their study (Goertzel & Goertzel, 1965) on the childhoods of persons of 'eminence', a characteristic defined as becoming 'important enough to their contemporaries to have books written about them':

> *there is a love of learning in one or both parents, often accompanied by a physical exuberance and a persistent drive toward goals.*

... the child who is both intelligent and creative remains society's most valuable resource ... his talents may reward us in ways beyond our ability to imagine.

Progress is not, however, inevitable. Prejudice and untruth run through the construct like geological fault-lines. There are chaotic eddies: pestilence, war and famine. In an evocative and sickening account of man's inhumanity and barbarism (Van Ee & Kleber, 2012), an aspect of humankind in the modern day is described: rape as a weapon of war and subjugation, with the children born of rape themselves at risk:

> *'Anselme is like a shadow,' Arya said, 'a shadow of the past that will haunt me forever.'*
>
> *... together they tried to reframe Anselme's life from rape-born to God-given.*

The template, though overtly permissive and 'open'-upwards, is also restrictive and constraining from below. 'Culture' has a pervasive dampening effect. There is an entrenched resistance to paradigm shifts. Suddenness of change is associated with unease, stress and instability. The determination that a planetary system is heliocentric rather than geocentric may be interpreted – bizarrely to us – as heresy. The time increments for cultural sway (as well as childhood mortality) are probably generational, not sudden.

Part of the stratal template is our literary and artistic heritage; in short, the stories we tell our children. These are fundamental to development, core values, perceived history, and from these: nature and identity. Our species has a long childhood (Bjorklund, 2007) to toy with stories. If we want to stoke the coals of nationalism, we should teach our children about brave freedom fighters and wars of independence, with field trips to sites of national triumph; show them swords and armour and forget cultural or social achievements and the trappings of civilisation. How much does the Scottish independence movement owe to early viewings of *Braveheart*?

Michael Rosen reviewed his time as Children's Laureate (Rosen, 2009), describing a disconnect between the UK politics of education and what a real education could be:

> *I say what's going on is discriminatory. Children who come from homes where books are being read get access to the kinds of abstract and complex ideas that you can only get hold of easily through exposure to extended prose. The rest are being fed worksheets.*

He also describes children's reactions to Capa's photographs of refugees fleeing in the Spanish Civil War (Rosen, 2009). He feels 'privileged' to sit in that space to talk and write about experiences of loss, real and imagined – of memories one would treasure if 'we had to leave home at a time of disaster'.

Rosen describes childhood as being (Kellaway, 2002) 'the place in which you "make" yourself'. When he is accused of being a 'grown-up child', he says:

> From the outside I may look childlike or childish because I have enthusiasms. I get engaged in the world. I can see some people think: look why don't you sort of just settle down?

Even as I read the article, and having read a few of Rosen's books, I want to insert a handwritten, smudged but legible, blue-ink 'refused to' between the typescript of the title 'The children's poet who' and 'grew up'. And leave 'grew' as 'grew'.

END AT THE BEGINNING

It has been a quiet Saturday morning in the Emergency Department. The 'Q' word is banned here because of the unhappy superstition, analogous to the commentator's curse, that it invites calamity. Anything can happen and it does: there is commotion on the ramp, two ambulance men shouting: 'Child – boy. Four years old. Pedestrian, hit by car. Unconscious, cervical collar. Fractured femur, splinted.'

We are ready: I am 'A & B'. This is what you train for. Blood, mud and dust are slaked down his side and torn shirt. His neck has a collar (*C-spine stabilised*), and he is on a spinal board. There is blood down his jeans and his leg is splinted. *Ignore it: focus on the airway and breathing, stratify, look for life-threatening injuries.* My left hand gently cups the back of his skull; his position is 'sniffing' already. I drop my turned head to 5 cm from his: *do you feel his breath on your cheek?* (No – not yet.)

Look south – watch for his chest moving. Is it moving? (No – not yet.) *Keep looking.* Still crouched, watching and feeling, I move my right hand towards his right arm: *find the brachial pulse.* Pippa, a nurse my age, is 'C', already bent over him from the far side, her tourniquet on his arm, tapping for a vein. We learn the ABC of resuscitation (Airway-Breathing-Circulation) as a sequence but, in practice, with multiple players, everything happens at once. Before my right hand reaches his elbow, I understand that everything is wrong: in the palm of my left hand, at the back of his head, above the collar, nothing is sensible.

I turn to look and withdraw my hand an inch. There is that moment of mutual understanding between the four of us: me, Pippa and the two ambulance men. We register the skull fragments and mashed brains, cupped in my hand: all that was identity, dripping through my fingers. The end.

We pause before lifting the blanket over his body and face, and I hear the mother's long, low howl from the ramp.

Later, in the 'Relatives' Room', I sit in front of her. She still clings to her shopping basket with a punctured football crammed in the top. Between sobs, she tells me about the accident, and about her boy. And I listen.

REFERENCES AND FURTHER READING

Bell S.W., McLaughlin D., Huntley J.S. Paediatric forearm fractures in the west of Scotland. *Scot. Med. J.* 2012; *57*(3): 139–43.

Bjorklund D.F. *Why youth is not wasted on the young: Immaturity in human development.* Malden, MA, Oxford and Melbourne: Blackwell Publishing; 2007.

Borges J.L. The garden of forking paths. In: *Labyrinths.* London: Penguin; 1970, pp. 44–53.

Brazelton T.B., Tronick E., Adamson L., et al. Early mother–infant reciprocity. *Ciba Found. Symp.* 1975; *33*: 137–54.

Center on the Developing Child, Harvard University. *The science of neglect: The persistent absence of responsive care disrupts the developing brain.* Working Paper No. 12. 2012. Available at: http://developingchild.harvard.edu/resources/reports_and_working_papers/working_papers/wp12/ (accessed 9 August 2015).

Center on the Developing Child, Harvard University. *In brief: The science of neglect* [video]. Cambridge, MA: Center on the Developing Child; 2015. Available at: http://developingchild.harvard.edu/resources/multimedia/videos/inbrief_series/inbrief_neglect/ (accessed 9 August 2015).

Court-Brown C.M., McBirnie J. The epidemiology of tibial fractures. *J. Bone Joint Surg. Br.* 1995; *77*(3): 417–21.

Eunson P. Learning from low income countries: What are the lessons? Communities should decide priorities. *BMJ.* 2004; *329*(7475): 1183.

Eunson P.D. Development: Are slogans appropriate? *Lancet.* 1984; *2*(8410): 1041–2.

Goertzel V., Goertzel M.G. Out of the cradle endlessly rocking. In: *Cradles of eminence.* London: Constable; 1965, pp. 271–93.

Harari Y.N. And they lived happily ever after. In: *Sapiens: A brief history of humankind.* London: Harvill Secker; 2014, pp. 376–96.

Horton R. Offline: Four drowning children. *Lancet.* 2015; *386*(9990): 230.

Horton R. Offline: Neurons, neighbourhoods, and the future for children. *Lancet.* 2013; *382*(9894): 754.

Huntley J.S. The Hunterian museum (Glasgow). *Scott. Med. J.* 2012; *57*(1): 1–3.

Huntley J.S. Traction and the Thomas splint. In: Carachi R., Agarwala S., Bradnock T.J., eds. *Basic techniques in paediatric surgery: An operative manual.* Berlin: Springer-Verlag; 2013, pp. 101–4.

Kavanagh R.G., Kelly J.C., Kelly P.M., et al. 2013. The 100 classic papers of pediatric orthopaedic surgery: A bibliometric analysis. *J. Bone Joint Surg. Am.* 2013; *95*(18): e134(1–8).

Kellaway K. The children's poet who grew up. *Guardian.* 27 October 2002. Available at: www.theguardian.com/books/2002/oct/27/poetry.features (accessed 3 August 2015).

Kipling R. If. In: *Rewards and fairies.* New York: Doubleday, Page & Company; 1910.

Larkin P. This be the verse. In: *High windows.* London: Faber & Faber; 1974.

Livingstone T. *Child of our time*: Whatever happened to our children's playtime? *Telegraph.* 31 May 2008. Available at: www.telegraph.co.uk/news/uknews /2059471/Child-Of-Our-Time-Whatever-happened-to-our-childrens -playtime.html (accessed 4 August 2015).

McDermott C., Quinlan J.F., Kelly I.P. Trampoline injuries in children. *J. Bone Joint Surg. Br.* 2006; *88*(6): 796–8.

Matthews T.J., Hamilton B.E. *Delayed childbearing: More women are having their first child later in life.* NCHS Data Brief No. 21. August 2009. Available at: www.cdc .gov/nchs/data/databriefs/db21.pdf (accessed 12 June 2015).

Mesman J., Van Ijzendoorn M.H., Bakermans-Kranenburg M.J. The many faces of the still-face paradigm: A review and meta-analysis. *Dev. Rev.* 2009; *29*(2): 120–62.

Newton I. Letter to Robert Hooke. 5 February 1676.

Rabinovitch D. Author of the month: Michael Rosen. *Guardian.* 24 November 2004. Available at: www.theguardian.com/books/2004/nov/24/booksforchi ldrenandteenagers.dinarabinovitch (accessed 3 August 2015).

Robertson E. *The Yorkhill story: The history of the Royal Hospital for Sick Children, Glasgow.* Glasgow: Yorkhill and Associated Hospitals Board of Management; 1972.

Rogers E.M. Elements of diffusion. In: *Diffusion of innovations.* 5th ed. New York: Free Press; 2003, pp. 1–38.

Rosen M. The ups and downs of a story. *Guardian.* 9 June 2009. Available at: www.theguardian.com/education/2009/jun/09/michael-rosen-creativity-in -the-classroom-teaching (accessed 3 August 2015).

Rosling H. The joy of facts and figures by Fiona Fleck. *Bull. World Health Organ.* 2013; *91*(12): 904–5.

Rosling H., Zhang Z. Health advocacy with Gapminder animated statistics. *J. Epidemiol Glob. Health.* 2011; *1*(1): 11–14.

Schaffer H.R. *Introducing child psychology.* Oxford: Blackwell Publishing; 2004.

Shonkoff J.P., Phillips D.A., eds. *From neurons to neighbourhoods: The science of early childhood development.* Washington, DC: National Academy Press; 2000.

Singer P. Famine, affluence, and morality. *Philos Public Affairs.* 1972; *1*(3): 229–43.

Singer P. The drowning child and the expanding circle. *New Internationalist.* April 1997.

Taylor-Whiffen P. *Interview with Professor Robert Winston, presenter of* Child of Our Time. Open University; 2005. Available at: https://view.officeapps.live .com/op/view.aspx?src=http%3A%2F%2Fwww3.open.ac.uk%2Fevents%2F7 %2F2005112_38827_o1.doc (accessed 3 August 2015).

Tronick E. *Still face experiment.* 2015. Available at: www.youtube.com/watch?v =apzXGEbZht0 (accessed 9 August 2015).

Tronick E., Als H., Adamson L., et al. The infant's response to entrapment between contradictory messages in face-to-face interaction. *J. Am. Acad. Child. Psych.* 1978; *17*(1): 1–13.

UNICEF. Child poverty in perspective: An overview of child well-being in rich countries. *Innocenti Report Card 7.* Florence: UNICEF Innocenti Research Centre; 2007.

UNICEF. Child well-being in rich countries: A comparative overview. *Innocenti report card 11.* Florence: UNICEF Office of Research; 2011.

Van Ee E., Kleber R.J. Child in the shadowlands. *Lancet.* 2012. *380*(9842): 642–3.

Wedge P., Prosser H. *Born to fail? The National Children's Bureau reports on striking differences in the lives of British children.* London: Arrow Books; 1973.

Winston R. 2006. Filming child development. *Observer.* January 2006. Available at: www.researchgate.net/profile/Robert_Winston/publication/275484429 _Filming_Child_Development/links/553dd52e0cf2c415bb0f79d6?origin =publication_list (accessed 4 August 2015).

6

STORY AS PERFORMANCE

Jacques Kerr and Colin Robertson

*An actor, like any other artist, is someone who can't forget. A painter's
medium is paint, a writer's words. An actor's medium is character.*

Callow, 1995

Public fascination with medicine is evident in the sheer number of
films, television and radio series, medical 'soaps' and reality shows.
Many healthcare professionals avoid watching these programmes.
They are too close to their daily life. But the interest is unsurprising.
Medicine encompasses and highlights every aspect of the human condition. It tells the best, most varied stories, heartwarming and uplifting
or tragic and saddening; every facet of human nature is brought to the
fore when individuals are sick or injured.

Acting is, however, more than mere entertainment. Whether we
are aware of it or not, performance is a foundation of our profession. Often without realising, clinicians are really actors who rehearse,
deliver scripts, modify their body language and subtly modulate vocal
tones on an intimate stage. Many doctors baulk at this idea. They perceive 'acting' as make-believe, pretence, play-acting, that is irrelevant
to clinical practice. The best clinical communicators, however, achieve
their goals, often unconsciously, by getting into a character part that
most effectively enables them.

THE HISTORICAL LINK BETWEEN
DRAMA AND MEDICINE

Performance has probably always accompanied healing. From the
earliest times, shamans used brightly coloured costumes and body

DOI: 10.1201/9781003409151-6

paint to channel spirits to enrich crops, enhance fertility and heal the sick. These rites still occur in the so-called 'primitive' tribes in the Amazon, Borneo and Australia. As with today's actors, a shaman's wardrobe and makeup are essential for the performance. With these tools, or props, there is not just communication, but transformation. Semiotically, exorcism for the possession by evil spirits is identical to the termination of seizure activity in a patient with status epilepticus.

In Ancient Greece, prayers were made to Asklepios, the god of medicine and healing. The prayers were thought to be answered in dreams describing cures and treatments for the ailment. The sufferer could also attend dramatic plays in the Asklepieion. Here they would watch their afflictions played out, leading to a resolution or *catharsis*. This technique was recognised in Aristotle's *Poetics*, the first real treatise on acting and literary theory. In this way, individuals could come to terms with the psychological elements of their illness. C S Lewis said 'we read to know that we are not alone' and it seems that hearing another human being tell their experience helps us and affirms our common identity. Nowadays, many of our patients, especially those with chronic or terminal diseases, obtain this contact, support and comfort through social media.

In Europe, these aspects began to take a back seat when, in the seventeenth century, the philosopher René Descartes postulated the notion of mind–body duality. The spiritual and philosophical aspects of this mind–body split are now largely discredited, but his thesis was instrumental in Western medicine developing along a path that emphasised physical cure, and ignoring or minimising the importance of the patient's spiritual and emotional needs. The doctor had become the God. As a result, practitioners were actively discouraged from incorporating the essential components of storytelling and drama in the healing process.

THE ACTING PROCESS

Acting is about finding and expressing dramatic truth. The best actors bring a story to life by embellishing a script, varying voice and movement, and making full and creative use of space. But, above all, the best actors hypnotise and bewitch by the unalloyed honesty of their portrayals. Emotional truth is the goal in acting and can only be achieved by avoiding mimickry, make-believe or play-acting.

Actors undergo intensive training in the disciplines of voice, movement, dance and stagecraft, very much in the same way that instrumentalists devote practice time to scales, technique, harmony and tone to conquer the psychomotor challenges of rendering a musical score. More importantly, musicians and actors strive to uncover the kernel of a work's identity; capturing a character's essence is at the heart of all good acting. But how one actor brings a character to life may be very different to how another takes on the same role – the creative putty is as unique as a fingerprint. This is not simply dependent on physicality; it is predicated primarily on a condensation of all the experience that has shaped that individual's identity up to that point. One flute player might play a Bach Andante with sorrow, whilst another expresses nostalgia; what determines each player's choice does not fall to their inner weather at that instant, but is based on a lifetime of experience and emotion.

Here we have an analogy to medical practice. Our approach to patients should be independent of how we feel at that moment; whether we've just had an argument with a colleague, been turned down for a job or even the happy obverse of finding out our partner is pregnant. When we engage with our patients it should be immaterial how we feel. Our approach must always be framed in empathy.

AN EXERCISE

'Ham acting' occurs when an emotion is expressed in a mechanistic, unbelieving way; the best acting draws on real emotions which the actor has experienced first-hand and uses to fuel their performance. In this respect, drama is a heightened, disciplined version of a behavioural process that clinicians perform daily, analogous to the relationship between an operatic performance and whistling an aria on your way to work. This does not mean that we should break down when imparting bad news, for example, but thinking and feeling ourselves into our patient's situation will invariably lead to a more empathic and supportive dialogue.

To illustrate, try a short exercise. Spend a few minutes immersing yourself in each of the following scenarios:

- You're in an interview for a medical job. It's not going well. You try to appear confident yet humble, knowledgeable yet deferential. You're aware that you are being studied and appraised. The interviewers throw you a curveball on a subject you know nothing about; your immediate reaction is one of blind fear and mental paralysis.

- Now imagine you're in a riverside pub. It's a glorious warm summer's evening, you're surrounded by your closest friends and family, the wine flows as freely as the anecdotes. It's idyllic, timeless, childlike, golden.
- Now you're in the middle of a blazing argument with your partner. You'd agreed that he would uproot and relocate so that you could take a promotion. You had discussed this, at length, and agreed that although it would involve sacrifice on his part it would be better for you both in the long run. But now he's changed his mind. He refuses to come. You are accused of being egocentric and ignoring his needs and his career.

Think of *who* you are in each situation. Think of your inner act; think of which aspects of your personality are being emphasised in each circumstance. Each scenario features you as protagonist, but the character you 'play' is subtly different. Certainly, at no point are you pretending or play-acting; you've simply chosen to express aspects of your personality that best suit the situation you're in, and, at the same time, to reject those that are irrelevant. This *is* acting by another name: professional acting simply formalises this technique of emphasising and de-emphasising the very different elements of our personalities for entertainment, therapy, role play or life coaching.

And so it is in other professions besides acting; the High Court judge during the day is a very different man to his infant grandchild when he goes home that evening. The Head of Surgical Services in a teaching hospital becomes a very different woman when she puts on dance shoes for her Wednesday evening ballroom dance class. Multiple personae can jostle within us and co-exist without being irreconcilable or pathological. Indeed, 'acting' can now seem to be more about a 'natural selection' process that adapts our personalities best to any given situation.

Hamlet's speech to the players in Act III, Scene II is a wonderful summary of how to act, and was Shakespeare's coded plea to his own actors. Note that this speech is delivered in prose, not verse, to emphasise the need for abandoning any ham acting (see Box 6.1).

BOX 6.1

Hamlet.
Speak the speech, I pray you, as I pronounced it to you, trippingly on the tongue. But if you mouth it, as many of your players do, I had as lief the town crier spoke my lines. Nor do not saw the air too much with your hand thus, but use all gently, for in the very torrent, tempest, and (as I may say) whirlwind of passion, you must acquire and beget a temperance that may give it smoothness. Oh, it offends me to the soul to hear a robustious peri-wig-pated fellow tear a passion to tatters, to very rags, to split the ears of the groundlings, who for the most part are capable of nothing but inexplicable dumb-shows and noise. I would have such a fellow whipped for o'erdoing Termagant. It out-Herods Herod. Pray you, avoid it.

First player.
I warrant your honour.

Hamlet.
Be not too tame neither, but let your own discretion be your tutor. Suit the action to the word, the word to the action, with this special observance that you o'erstep not the modesty of nature. For anything so overdone is from the purpose of playing, whose end, both at the first and now, was and is to hold, as 'twere, the mirror up to nature, to show virtue her own feature, scorn her own image, and the very age and body of the time his form and pressure. Now this overdone or come tardy off, though it make the unskillful laugh, cannot but make the judicious grieve, the censure of the which one must in your allowance o'erweigh a whole theatre of others.

So how does an actor adopt an identity when playing a role? And how can they be themselves and someone else at the same time? Actors in rehearsal and performance will say that their character 'waits in the wings', simmering under the surface of who they are, ready to manifest when the lights go up. Musicians report that simply picking up their instrument, even before they begin to play, opens up the ideational wonderland. This is the creative state of Nirvana desired by all artists; they lose or suspend awareness of the passage of time; become fully focused, energised and enter a pleasurable zone labelled by Croatian psychologist Mihály Csíkszentmihályi as 'flow'. Many actors report that acting on a stage is the best feeling that they ever experience and that nothing comes close. Some clinicians experience something similar when carrying out a complex interventional procedure; an eight-hour operation may pass rapidly for the totally focused surgeon, while those leading resuscitation scenarios describe a similar phenomenon of suspension of time – hence a scribe is essential in charting the events.

From a psychological viewpoint, there is an analogy with how artists draw and paint realistically. Betty Edwards's book *Drawing on the Right Side of the Brain* proposed that we can only draw and paint effectively and with realism if we 'switch off' our dominant left hemisphere and engage the creative mode of the right. This was based on theories developed by Sperry and Gazzaniga that the two cerebral hemispheres have different modes of function; the left, devoted to language processing, is analytical, mathematical, reasons sequentially and is essentially convergent in its thinking; whereas the right hemisphere is global, synthetic, intuitive, imaginative and divergent. The book (and drawing courses) offers exercises to fast-track the ability of students to draw. Clark Bowlen argued for a similar split-brain model of how actors realise a role through housing the character in the 'creative' right hemisphere: 'Acting is a duality. It is being two persons at once. An actor does not just signify or depict a character, he truly becomes another person. Yet he remains himself. He is two realities in one.'

Current research suggests that the split-brain concept is incorrect; some brain functions do, indeed, occur in one hemisphere, but neuroimaging and EEG studies indicate that creativity, whether artistic or scientific, is not localised to one or other hemisphere or even within specific brain locations. There is no doubt, however, that many artists and performers have been energised by the idea. Perhaps its true value, however flawed neuroscientifically, is to stimulate and liberate new ways of approaching performance by giving individuals a forge in which to smelt the pertinent characteristics of their personalities to render a character.

Some individuals exemplify the synergy between art and medicine. Kate Bassett's biography of Jonathan Miller showcases the versatile genius of a man who was at one with the arts and medicine. An accomplished polymath, Sir Jonathan initially trained in medicine before being bitten by the drama bug and taking the highly unconventional and risqué *Beyond the Fringe* to Edinburgh in the 1960s. Building on his experience he forayed further into theatre and opera directing before creating the groundbreaking *The Body in Question,* a 13-part television series, which he wrote and presented (Figure 6.1). This explored all aspects of the history and philosophy of medicine, culminating in a cadaver dissection, which at the time drew criticism for being potentially distressing to some viewers. Sir Jonathan continued to spin the plates of acting and medicine throughout his life, finding strong and innovative links between the two and enriching both.

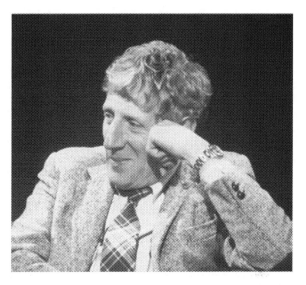

Figure 6.1 Jonathan Miller by Open Media Ltd. (Open Media Ltd, CC BY-SA 3.0, https://commons.wikimedia.org/w/index.php?curid=62888097)

BUILDING A CHARACTER

Much of modern acting theory and practice is based on the principles of Konstantin Stanislavski (1863–1938). He developed a *praxis* of acting that revolutionised how actors tackle the creating and actualising of a character. This brings together a number of strands that equip an actor with their role, including voice, movement and stagecraft, with the overarching aim that the actor achieves dramatic realism. Stanislavski emphasised the need for an actor to use their wealth of experience, emotional intelligence and kinaesthetic memory to fuel and bring a character to life. By doing so, the actor empowers the audience to suspend their disbelief and be immersed in the story; each audience member becomes a lie-detector who instinctively recognises and rejects portrayals that are not emotionally truthful.

More recently Lee Strasberg's 'method acting', the 'doctrine' taught in The Actors' Studio, a converted church sited in the Manhattan area of New York, has gained popularity. This sees the actor researching their character extensively, striving for truth and realism to the point that they actually live the experience, ensuring an imprinted and accurate emotional memory. The story of Dustin Hoffman subjecting himself to sleep deprivation for his character in *Marathon Man* is an extreme example (on hearing how he'd researched the role, his co-star, Sir Laurence Olivier, iconically responded, 'But why don't you just act it, dear boy?'). It is remarkable how many clinicians' views on analgesia, sedation and 'minor' procedures are dramatically changed once they have experienced the process themselves!

To unlock the relevant characteristics that constitute a character, the trained actor has a number of possible routes and different techniques. As with other creative professions, actors vary in which works best for them. Some respond best to 'animal work' – this relies on the assumption that every character can be likened to a specific animal; discovering which animal is the best 'fit' enables ready access to that character. Once the actor has decided on which particular animal best suits the character, he or she then studies this animal, in zoos, on programmes, in books and on the internet, to actualise its physicality kinaesthetically and to reproduce its soundscape through vocal modulation, to bring the same presence to the character. For example, Aleksandr Vershinin in Chekhov's *Three Sisters* might be played as a puppy, Iago in *Othello*, a snake, Caliban in *The Tempest*, a monkey.

Animal work, imitation of a friend's walk, costume-dressing, use of simple props and living the part, can all get an actor into character. These techniques help to dovetail their personality traits into those of the character. It is unlikely that any of us would have the opportunity to play the role of a serial killer, an eighteenth-century lady of the manor, a powerful genie or the captain of a sinking ship. However, we all have the capacity to *be* them and to find common traits and elements in our affective memories that express the essence of the character in question.

Extending these aspects into medicine may seem far-fetched, but building our character as doctors has strong resonance. The role of costume is just as relevant to medicine as it is to acting. When you put on your white coat, scrubs or uniform and drape a stethoscope around your neck or put on your mask, you are unconsciously performing the same process. Costume is a powerful lever in building our medical character. Even after studies demonstrated that infection was more likely to be transmitted by wearing anything below the elbow, white coats took years to shed because of their power to get us into character. Like it or not, our patients judge a book by its cover; they prefer a neatly groomed individual in traditional attire and white coat with a clearly legible name tag.

Children use costumes in dressing-up games; a police uniform or fireman's outfit grants permission to become that character and functions like a protective shell against disempowerment. For us, a surgical gown or uniform does more than protect against infection; it confers the right to operate and intervene. Even a surgical mask is about more than protection; it places the emphasis on the surgeon's eyes and de-emphasises the mouth – the story being told in this 'theatre' is not merely a spoken narrative.

However, this process can go awry. Actors sometimes fall prey to 'possession syndrome' – the character subsumes their identity and they lose the demarcation between their personality and the character they are playing. This can happen in medicine when our role takes over all we do and say and eclipses who we are as an individual. It is crucial for our well-being and mental health that we have dedicated time away from medicine: with our families and loved ones, enjoying sports and hobbies, ensuring our brains and bodies engage in non-medical pursuits.

An essential of acting training is to make us face our weaknesses; it is impossible to play a role if we are uncomfortable with a particular character trait. We will shy away from expressing this and our character will lose dimension and credibility. Playing a character who has a trait that we ourselves possess but are ashamed of, makes it impossible to bring that character to life. A character that is a homosexual will be impossible to play if we are uncomfortable with our own sexuality. Similarly, caring for a patient with traits that we despise in ourselves will make it difficult to relate to and empathise with that patient.

It takes a huge amount of affective memory to play a role. Actors constantly look out for experiences that will extend the range of their emotional palette. Simon Callow, in *Being an Actor*, tells of Michael MacLiammoir who, hearing that his best friend may have died, burst into tears and ran downstairs to the reception desk of the hotel he was staying in. On the way down he passed a mirror and caught sight of himself in it. 'Oh,' he thought, 'that's what one looks like when the person dearest to one in the whole world has just died.'

By analogy, to be an effective clinician also takes prodigious feats of memory: this is not simply the knowledge of the trade; it is about the huge range of characters we encounter. Reading a patient's character is as important in diagnosing and managing their clinical condition as knowledge of that condition. A stoical farmer who comes into the Emergency Department with severe abdominal pain and a history only of a hernia repair is a very different prospect to read from the teenage girl who denies ever having had sexual intercourse and presents with abdominal swelling and amenorrhoea.

REHEARSAL AND TEAM-PLAYING

Great performances make us feel that we are a fly on the wall, stealing a glimpse at a real-life situation. For the actor, this necessitates many hours of rehearsal. Only after much trial and error is the play finally transformed into a show fit for an audience. Even after the first night, the show has a life and natural history of its own. A drama is never crystallised, but remains organic throughout its run, mutating its identity from one night to the next, creating unpredictability and surprise with every line. Actors forget their lines, props fail, lights don't come up, the audience doesn't react in the expected way; these 'happy failures' challenge the actors to stay on their toes, keeping the performances alive and organic. Moreover, the play changes its character; actors find new meaning in their lines, bringing subtle shifts in the lens through which they view their characters. The knock-on effect is that the complex adaptive system of stageplay is altered, often with an unexpectedly good outcome.

The rehearsal process is as relevant, and unpredictable, in clinical practice. Medical students initially engage in rehearsal with their first patients. Most students have enough social confidence and life skills to speak easily with strangers, enquire about their health and well-being, and pass the time of day. But asked to take a history from a 70-year-old woman with heart failure, that skill and confidence vanishes. Partly, it is the lack of knowledge of what to ask and the significance of understanding what this relates to, but mainly the anxiety stems from the first foray into taking on a role that will be seen and audited by a foremost expert in medical 'behaviour', the patient. Patients are the ultimate lie-detectors, and children are the most discerning of all. Patients are highly knowledgeable, practised critics. Often they have seen hordes of aspiring medics during their personal journey of health and disease and can tell instantly whether a student or doctor knows what they're doing. This is why professional actors are increasingly used in under- and postgraduate medical examinations; all of us have been a patient at some time; the ex-patient who is also an actor is therefore the best assessor of all. Their professional acting training enables them to maintain a consistent response in any medical interrogation and to improvise as required.

From the practical viewpoint, drama school and medical school have very similar scholastic matrices with their attendant psychomotor, emotional and social challenges. The choreography of a laparoscopic cholecystectomy or cardiac arrest resuscitation closely resembles the complex interplay of the rehearsal room; the subtle difference is that the patient, as principal actor, has no conscious part to play in the drama. However, their unvoiced story continues to be told through their anatomy, physiology and response to therapy.

THE SCRIPT

Acting usually involves a script. Even if there are no spoken lines, the script suggests to the actor which movements to make, where and when to exit the stage, what props are needed, where the piece is set and other such logistic considerations. Similarly, a music score contains directions on how a piece should be played. In drama, directions may be open to interpretation, allowing the actor flexibility around who the character is; on the other hand, some scripts may be very well prescribed. All actors are familiar with the moment when script becomes living character; after weeks of learning their lines, they forge a connection with the text that is more than just declarative memory and take ownership so that the words become the very tissue that makes up the character. Shakespeare often takes great pains to direct the actor, even giving clues as to which animal the character would be: Iago's speeches have a repeated alveolar sibilant 'S' sound, signifying that the character should be portrayed as the archetypal serpent which poisons the mind of Othello against Desdemona.

Although not written down, a 'script' is equally necessary when communicating with patients and relatives. Sometimes the patient or relative will be on the same page of the script as you, will react in an expected way, give the appropriate cues and the scene will close with the objective having been accomplished cleanly. However, the well-documented sequence of emotional reactions (denial, anger, depression and acceptance) that individuals experience in a breaking-bad-news situation may not take place. They may react unpredictably and 'off book', necessitating improvisation.

Communication between healthcare professionals is often overlooked but also exists in a medium of narrative; the paramedic relays the 'story' to the emergency doctor or nurse who then hands over to the receiving physician. The junior doctor presents the patient to the consultant on the post-take ward round. How the story is told can take many forms, but increasingly there is an emphasis on a structured handover through an SBAR (Situation-Background-Assessment-Recommendation) approach.

STAGECRAFT AND THE PERFORMANCE SPACE

Regardless of whether a dramatic piece is set indoors, outdoors, in site-specific arenas or in the air, there is always a stage. Stagecraft is the technical process of bringing actors, scene changes, lighting and sound together onto a stage to create a whole. Stagecraft is implicit in many situations. Although we might not call it acting, there is an obvious performance drama in weddings or funerals, the christening of a child, the changing of the guard, the arrangement of a symphony orchestra, and the assembly of a court room. The actors' use of the stage is called *blocking*; depending on the director, the play and the actors (and the available space), actors may block out a piece at first rehearsal and adhere to these placings thereafter or, as is the case with, for example, Mike Leigh's work, the blocking may be actor-driven over the whole rehearsal period, where movements are determined by the emotion and action of the moment.

Different 'stages' have different layouts, but ultimately they share one common feature – positioning the key figure at centre stage; everything is arranged such that the spatial geometry optimises the power of the narrative. The summing-up speech in a trial by jury, the delivery of a sermon, the leading of a trauma resuscitation, all position the protagonist at a point that maximises their 'storytelling'. Acting within, and dictated by, the confines of a given space therefore has strong parallels with medical practice. Increasingly, we are aware of the relevance and importance of blocking in the design of our hospitals, wards and theatres and in the conduct of scenarios such as major trauma management, operative surgery and prehospital care. The arrangement of medical students, junior doctors, nursing staff and consultants on a medical ward round has a powerfully dramatic presence. In miniature, the crowding of the team around the patient's bed echoes the projection of the stage into the groundling's pit of Elizabethan theatres such as the Globe (Figure 6.2).

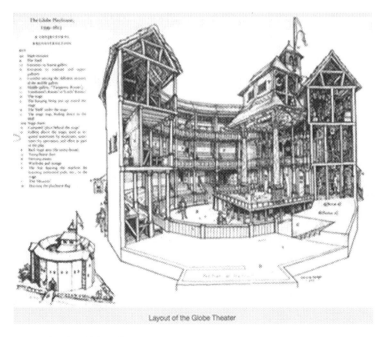

Figure 6.2 The Globe Theatre.

The use of 'props' on the medical 'stage' varies depending on situation and requirement. Props are obviously crucial in operating theatres, interventional radiology suites and even the business post-take ward round where the humble stethoscope makes a frequent appearance – although perhaps not as often as it should. In some cases the prop may actually be the principal actor, such as in the use of robotic surgery. When doctors have to convey information or break bad news, props should be minimal; for example, the doctor should not carry a pager or phone to ensure that there is no disturbance. With the exception of items that the relatives might need, e.g. a box of tissues and a glass of water, this situation is often more 'anti-prop'. And where behaviour is concerned, the clinician needs to use the correct 'character' to communicate; voices should be quietened, movements and information delivered slowly, clearly and unambiguously without jargon.

Stagecraft is central to the delivery of medical teaching. Lectures are perfect examples of an educational drama where the student audience attends a one-person play for an hour or two at a time. It is an often-held fallacy that lectures are boring and dry. Some lecturers are natural actors who bring vitality and verve to their teaching, often inducing the switch from 'left to right brain' in their audience so that the whole experience is timeless. And storytelling features strongly in this context; we often remember an entertaining anecdote clearly as an illustration of the educational point.

It is interesting to note that in a lecture setting, the slides are not so much prompts as props; line-prompting in a theatre kills the flow and energy of the piece as does reading the bullet points of a slide. The best lecturers use teaching aids as props – similar to an actor using visual cues around the stage to remind him of his next line or move.

By contrast, tutorials have more precise, intimate stagecraft. There are two different types of tutorial: closed and open. In a *closed* tutorial, information is imparted, almost didactically, but with the expectation that the tutees have read the subject and are in a position to answer posited questions; for example, the interpretation of blood abnormalities, or the conducting system of the heart; there is an established body of knowledge and the tutorial setting is used as a forum to talk over examples, give clinical settings and so on. In this situation, there is a script that is closely followed; the tutor is director, writer and author of what lies under discussion; her knowledge is uncontested.

In the *open* tutorial, the tutor is facilitator and arbiter; their role is to guide, steer and act as a conduit. Subjects under discussion in these situations might be:

- Should relatives be allowed into a resuscitation room during the management of a cardiac arrest?
- Is it legally and ethically acceptable to prescribe contraception to a girl who is 'underage'?
- Is it reasonable to break the bad news of an individual's death via telephone if the relative lives many miles away?

Here, there are no 'right' answers. There is greater latitude around how the issue will be discussed and a much higher possibility of free-fall, depending on the experience, beliefs and often strongly held views of the tutees.

The seating arrangement in each type of tutorial can support the style of the discussion; closed tutorials, arranged like mini-proscenium arch lectures with the students occupying a C position around the tutor; open tutorials, in the round, the tutor taking up an equal position with the students (Figure 6.3).

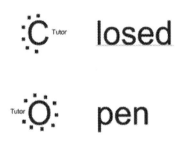

Figure 6.3 Closed and open tutorial settings.

SO WHAT CAN ACTING TEACH MEDICINE?

There are clearly strong parallels between medicine and acting. Training equips actors to withstand the onslaught of playing the same role whilst remaining refreshed and rejuvenated after every performance. We can annex many of these techniques to our, and our patients' and colleagues', advantage. It is clearly inappropriate to send doctors to drama school, but there is real scope in giving doctors some foundation in the training of acting to equip them for what lies ahead in their careers. Some courses see students spending time working as auxiliary nurses; this gives them an insight into the nurse's role and engenders respect and understanding for our colleagues.

In our post-COVID19 world, public perceptions have changed markedly and patients and their relatives are more sighted than ever on their interactions with the medical workforce. The majority of complaints are not about mistakes or medical negligence but about staff attitude.

The ideal doctor is expected to be continually empathic but, faced with yet another demanding patient, how can anyone expect to have unlimited reserves of compassion and care, especially for someone they've never met and may have nothing in common with? Occasionally, actors fall prey to the same syndrome by expecting to feel something every time they do a cold reading. No amount of acting training can manufacture an emotion unless we use character as a conduit and, as doctors, the process of building a character is essential to maintaining empathy. This is distinct from learning and repeating a 'script' with which we have no emotional connection. At heart, doctors, like actors, are trying to understand and communicate the human condition.

REFERENCES AND FURTHER READING

Aristotle. *Poetics*. Heath M., trans. London: Penguin; 1996.

Attenborough R., dir. *Shadowlands* [film]. Nicholson W., writer. 1993.

Au S., Khandwala F., Stelfox H.T. Physician attire in the intensive care unit and family perceptions of physician professional characteristics. *JAMA Intern. Med.* 2013; *173*(6): 465–7.

Baile W.F., Buckman R., Lenzi R., et al. SPIKES – A six-step protocol for delivering bad news: Application to the patient with cancer. *Oncologist.* 2000; *5*(4): 302–11.

Bowlen C. A right brain/left brain model of acting. Paper presented at the Annual Meeting of the American Theatre Association, Toronto, Canada, 4–7 August 1985.

Callow S. *Being an actor*. Revised ed. London: Penguin; 1995.

Dietrich A., Kanso R. A review of EEG, ERP, and neuroimaging studies of creativity and insight. *Psychol. Bull.* 2010; *136*(5): 822–48.

Edwards B. *Drawing on the right side of the brain: A course in enhancing creativity and artistic confidence*. London: HarperCollins; 2001.

Gurr A., Ichikawa M. *Staging in Shakespeare's theatres*. Oxford: Oxford University Press; 2000.

Hartigan K.V. *Performance and cure: Drama and healing in Ancient Greece and contemporary America*. London: Duckworth; 2009.

Lill M.M., Wilkinson T.J. Judging a book by its cover: Descriptive survey of patients' preferences for doctors' appearance and mode of address. *BMJ.* 2005; *331*(7531): 1524–7.

Nielsen J.A., Zielinski B.A., Ferguson M.A., et al. An evaluation of the left-brain vs. right-brain hypothesis with resting state functional connectivity magnetic resonance imaging. *PLOS ONE.* 2013; *8*(8): e71275.

Shakespeare W. *Hamlet*. 2nd revised ed. Jenkins H., ed. The Arden Shakespeare. Lindon: Bloomsbury Publishing PLC; 1999.

Stanislavski K. *Building a character*. London: Methuen Drama; first published 1950, reprinted 1997.

Zucker C. *In the company of actors: Reflections on the craft of acting*. London: A&C Black; 1999.

7

A STUDENT'S STORY

Sarah Richardson and Colin Robertson

My earliest memories are fragmentary. It is common not to be able to recall exact details or facts, but a narrative of specific events is common, often reinforced by repetition and corroboration from family and friends. The information has been contextualised and is therefore retrievable. Our development of language at around two to three years allows competent storage and processing of memories. Now, for the first time, I can express a timeline.

Intrinsic to developing narrative are false stories. Children from the age of three can, and do, lie. It is fundamental to their understanding of the story process and of their language ability. The reason may be to avoid the consequence of an action, to impress, manipulate or exaggerate. But, at least in part, it enables them to explore or analyse the response. For the first time, the child now knows that their thoughts and feelings are unique to themselves. They cannot be mind-read, and this offers clear opportunities. Aesop's fable of the boy that cried 'Wolf', and George Washington and his father's cherry tree are adult cautionary attempts in story form to educate the child to think twice before being deceitful. There is debate as to whether this technique is effective and, given the current scarcity of wolves, hatchets and accessible cherry trees, there may be a need to update these tales.

For my third birthday I received a toy doctor's kit. I asked my mother 'What do doctors do?' She said, 'If you are poorly, you may need to see a doctor. A doctor will try to help you get better.' A two-sentence story: Characters; Problem; Resolution; simple enough for me to understand but fundamental. The story gave a platform on which I could build that particular aspect of my knowledge. Parental influences aside, for many, TV shows and movies are often central to

DOI: 10.1201/9781003409151-7

the decision to become a doctor. *Holby City*, *ER* and *Casualty* certainly influenced me. The excitement and background stories are enticing, while many characters are good role models. Memories of Doctor Carter performing solo thoracotomies, making surgical airways with a biro and burr holes to decompress head injuries in the *ER*, certainly influenced and attracted me. The question of whether the authenticity of fictional medical stories affects our perception, and hence our choices, is more worrying. Take, for example, the ultimate medical emergency – cardiac arrest. In the UK, overall survival rates following out-of-hospital cardiac arrest are approximately 8–10% with 75–95% of cases having a primary cardio-respiratory cause. In one study of US TV programmes, the commonest cause of the arrest was trauma (gunshot, road accidents, drowning, electrocution) and the overall hospital discharge rate following CPR was 67% (Diem et al., 1996). A recent study of 70 fictional TV cardiac arrests portrayed an initial survival rate of 46%, the average age of the 'patients' was 36 years and cardio-respiratory causes were a minor group (Harris and Willoughby, 2009). As a consequence, and unsurprisingly, secondary-school students who watch TV medical 'soaps' significantly overestimate the chances of CPR success (Van den Bulck, 2002).

Everyone's first patient story is unique and unforgettable. TV soaps, and repeatedly reading my first-aid manual, were little preparation. Only as a teenage first-aider did I start to understand the concept of treating a patient. I was at a fair in my hometown and a young girl was brought to my first-aid post. It was my turn, and my stomach flipped at the thought of putting my training into practice. She had a twisted ankle, something I now see ten times a day at work but which, at the time, seemed pretty scary. She was clearly in pain and struggled to weight bear. I took a basic history and examined her, but was really none the wiser as to what was wrong or whether it was serious or trivial. The senior medic in the first-aid post was a doctor. In minutes, he established all the information I had missed, examined the ankle, excluded the need for X-ray, gave RICE advice and discharged her with her parents. After she left, he explained the common mechanisms of ankle injury, the basis of the Ottawa ankle rules and treatment options. I still recall the rules because of that.

MEDICAL SCHOOL: STARTING OUT

What is most difficult about going to medical school is the transition from the spoon-fed information process at secondary school to attending lectures and needing to do several further hours of study to even make sense of the information that you have been given. During the first weeks it is easy to become completely overwhelmed by the sheer quantity of information. As a result, fresher students seek guidance from their superiors throughout the medical school to find out the best ways to study.

Because of our hard-wired nature for narrative, a 'How and Why' is the mechanism we most commonly use to remember and assimilate information. When there is a need to override this, for example when lists of isolated facts need to be memorised, the process is much more difficult. We are poorly designed to retain non-contextualised information. No matter how slowly and clearly you speak, without a narrative to give framework and purpose I am unlikely to retain what you tell me. Undergraduate medicine, and its examination structure, is packed with the need to recall this type of information often as lists: the causes of finger clubbing, the sequence and names of the cranial nerves, the drugs used to treat hypertension. For some students, a mnemonic, acrostic or acronym may make the sequence 'memorable', but this is unreliable and only about 20% of students use these methods frequently (Brotle, 2011). For most, it is the combination of the story and physically seeing a condition or physical sign that is necessary to 'cement' the lesson.

BOX 7.1 'GETTING THROUGH FIRST YEAR'

A few weeks into first year we had an unusual lecture. A second-year medical student was introduced, stood up and simply told us his story.

At school he had 'aced' every exam; achieved straight-A passes in all his leavers' exams. He had sailed his way to medical school and came to first year certain of continuing success. He attended most lectures and tutorials but had not done much outside the set course. He sat his exams with confidence and proceeded to fail them all.

He looked at us. He reminded us that everyone in that lecture theatre was an A-grade student. We had already clearly proven that we had some level of intelligence. At school, that was often sufficient for success. But intelligence without application was no longer an option. He hadn't realised the quantity of work required, and had been complacent and over-confident. He predicted (and was correct) that significant numbers of us would drop out that year, not because the work was too challenging or conceptually difficult, but because the motivation to be there was not their own or because they had no desire to work. We all had ability, but the good students are those who really want to use it for the right reasons.

We sat silently for a minute after he stopped speaking. For many, his story was a spur to help cope in the seemingly interminable jungle of physiology, anatomy and biochemistry of those early years.

What was the most interesting lecture you attended, what made it special? We spend over 15,000 hours of structured education at school and a further 5,000 at medical school. But how many classes or tutorials can you really remember? Probably, only three or four. Understanding why so many are unmemorable is the key to improving the student's, and trainee's, experience. Here are two examples that illustrate different ways of engaging a student in the patient's story.

BOX 7.2 'LIVING' THE PATIENT'S STORY

It's a wild generalisation, but many students find it difficult to relate to the elderly and their conditions. When you are young, fit and active, frailty, incontinence and the intricacies of daily living are not as exciting as say, major trauma, transplantation and intricate interventional radiology. Accordingly, the tutorial on 'Common fractures in the elderly' was not awaited with great interest. The orthopaedic registrar tried hard. She took us to see Miss Sievewright, an elderly lady with a Colles' fracture. The X-rays and description of the reduction technique were moderately interesting, but our interest flagged. During the explanation of the after-care needed, she saw me yawn.

'Have *you* ever had a fracture or a cast on a limb?'
'No.'
'Do you want to feel what it is like?'
'OK.'
'Are you right-handed?
'Very.'

The registrar supervised my classmate's inexpert application of a plaster of Paris backslab to my right wrist and forearm. The cast felt heavy but the warm sensation as it dried was curiously comforting.

'Why not see what it's like to wear it and tell us tomorrow,' she said, and I went home proudly exhibiting my cast. I was 'living' a common orthopaedic story – albeit without the associated pain and swelling.

Problems started immediately. I struggled to turn the doorknob to my room and nearly dropped the kettle when making coffee. Worse, I couldn't toilet myself properly or dress – if you don't believe me, just you try washing, doing up a back-fastening bra, wiping your bum or tying trainer laces with your non-dominant hand. It was deeply, deeply humiliating.

Next day the registrar removed my sorry, soiled cast. It was a relief.

'You're lucky,' she said. 'You're healthy, pain-free and young. Miss Sievewright isn't. She lives alone. She will be in a cast for six weeks. Her orthopaedic story is really just starting.'

BOX 7.3 'DOCTOR, I WANT A BABY'

What, in other hands, might have been a dry, factual presentation was transformed by one obstetrician. He interweaved the physiology and anatomy of infertility with their accompanying treatment options with stories of women with different underlying conditions who presented to the clinic.

'I've been trying for two years, something must be wrong.'
'I have PCOS, what can you do to help me have a baby?'
'I'm 37 years old. What are the chances of something going wrong?'

The facts were all there, but contextualised, they became vivid and meaningful. This could be me. It was such a simple method for passing information on to students, but five years later, I still remember the content.

OTHER CULTURES, OTHER STORIES

Student electives can be life-changing. I had dreamt of going to Africa almost as long as I had of being a doctor. After much deliberation I decided on Tanzania. There, I could both work and indulge my love of the outdoors and trekking. I contacted a volunteering organisation online and had the choice of an urban placement close to the foothills of Mount Kilimanjaro or a rural placement in the southwest. I chose Mpanda District Hospital in the southern Rukwa region, 1,200 km from Dar es Salaam.

The journey took six days, with a day on the Zambian border, an eight-hour 300 km bus ride and hitch-hiking with Arab gem miners for the final 240 km of dirt road to the hospital.

I shadowed Dr Salum, an Assistant Medical Officer (AMO – a two-year diploma qualification that allows for the practice of basic medicine) and Dr Chaote, the one qualified doctor practising in the hospital. Before the morning outpatient clinic, we toured the hospital's six wards, two theatres, matron's office, the kitchens and the laundry and met every member of staff. The numbers of patients waiting to be assessed in the clinic were staggering (Figure 7.1).

My first patient walked in with a limp and multiple bandages poorly wrapped around both legs. Musa was around 60 years old, though most rural Africans do not know their birth date and count the number of harvests to approximate their age. I knew little Swahili at the time, so Dr Salum translated. Musa had had leg ulcers for several months and

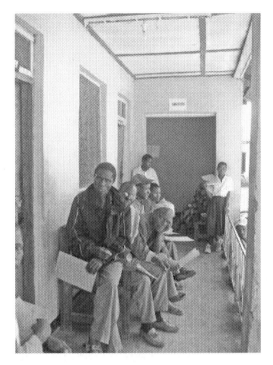

Figure 7.1 Outpatients at Mpanda District Hospital.

was in significant constant pain. He had had several courses of 'basic' antibiotics, but none had worked. The ulcers were getting bigger, deeper and more painful. Now he was unable to work in the fields to support his family. Dr Salum explained that once tropical ulcers were established, they required antibiotic and anti-fungal combinations and a complex dressing regimen. Musa bowed his head. He said '*sina pesa kwangu*': 'I have no money, my family is poor.' He looked up and we had eye contact for several seconds, then he sighed, looked away, thanked us both and took a prescription for all that he could afford – another basic, but cheap, antibiotic.

Over the next few months, I learnt the workings of the hospital. I gained a basic understanding of complex tropical diseases such as malaria, typhoid, cholera and hepatitis – diseases that I would never see at home. In the HIV/AIDS and TB clinics, I heard the stories behind the spread of these diseases in the region. The grandmother who brought six grandchildren to the clinic for check-ups; three had HIV and one had progressed to AIDS. Their parents had died of AIDS-related illnesses several years ago. She held the burden of the care of her grandchildren entirely alone. She explained that she had

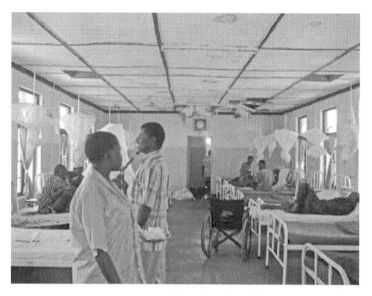

Figure 7.2 Male surgical ward at Mpanda District Hospital.

gone back to work to pay for food; she couldn't afford to send the children to school all the time, but the two 'well' children sometimes went if she could find the money to pay for books and uniforms.

These were powerful, touching individual stories. Although initially overwhelmed, with each one I gained a little more insight into their lives, increased my understanding of basic diagnostics and disease management, and became increasingly aware of my sheltered and privileged upbringing.

Because the hospital was so rural, it lacked many resources. Blood tests were limited, the ultrasound machine was faulty and power to supply the X-ray machine and theatres was intermittent. Stocks of medications would run low, necessitating rationing of 'precious' drugs such as diazepam for tetanus and opioids for trauma. I thought that managing some conditions without the most basic of resources was impossible, but the staff repeatedly told me stories of patients cured using only anxiolytics or 'antique' antibiotic regimens.

BACK TO THE FUTURE

My transition back to Western medicine was much more difficult than I had anticipated. I was in the Emergency Department of a major teaching hospital, as full of patients and relatives as Mpanda's had been, but oh, how different.

A patient had been referred with a wound infection after recent surgery. He had waited a couple of hours and it was clear that he was unhappy. The consultant introduced himself and explained that I would sit in on the consultation. The patient remained silent; when asked about the current problem he launched into an aggressive speech about long waiting times, lack of care from his GP, inappropriate waits for tests to be completed and a general attack on the doctors, nurses and the NHS.

I was taken aback. I'd always had the impression that it was the Friday night drunk patients that were aggressive, not a middle-aged man on a Monday afternoon.

The consultant calmly apologised for the waiting time, explained there had been a number of emergencies and that they were doing the best they could. The patient was not placated. He continued to complain about poor levels of care. After further apologies, the consultant suggested that they deal with his medical issue. In fact, the wound infection was minor and required an additional antibiotic course. He was discharged as disgruntled as he had arrived.

I was baffled by the patient's self-righteousness, arrogance and aggression. I had just come from Tanzania where I'd seen a woman walk 84 km in two days to hand over her dying child for assessment which then cost her money. I struggled with the concept that anyone could accuse the NHS of a substandard level of care. This man had attended a free GP appointment for a complication following free surgery for a chronic non–life-threatening issue and within three hours in an Emergency Department had a nursing assessment, blood tests and wound swabs, assessment with a specialist and a course of antibiotics, all for free.

Over coffee I expressed this forcibly to the consultant. 'You only know a small part of his story,' he said. 'Perhaps his wife has just left him, maybe he has a sick child at home. Perhaps his job is at risk if he doesn't get back to work.' He explained that there is no point arguing with these patients; they don't have an understanding of the pressures the staff working at the hospital are under or their stories. 'Choose your battles,' he said.

WE CAN KEEP LEARNING FROM STORIES

Every day patients surprise us. Sometimes they get sicker despite everything we do. Sometimes they die when we don't expect it. Sometimes we miss clues and get things wrong, but get away with it; sometimes we don't.

Jen was in her mid-twenties, completely fit and well up until a few days before she attended. I picked up her notes, sighed, and said to the nurses, 'She really should have just seen her GP.'

'I've come because I can't run up a hill properly any more.' She was a hill runner and regularly ran marathons in under three hours. She'd tried running for the past three days but became tired and breathless. She had a slight niggle in the right side of the chest but no specific symptoms. Observations were normal, oxygen saturations 98%, a respiratory rate of 16 and heart rate of 80 bpm. A quick set of bloods, a D-dimer and a chest X-ray seemed a little excessive but wouldn't do any harm. I sent her to sit and await the results. Half an hour later I was called to find her collapsed in the waiting room. In the resuscitation room, her BP and oxygen saturations were dangerously low, the heart rate was through the roof. Something had gone badly wrong.

With IV fluids, oxygen, a thrombolytic and ventilation she improved enough to make it up to ICU. The CT confirmed that the thrombus had fragmented distally in the pulmonary tree. After a stormy month, she was well enough for rehabilitation.

I tell her story to my students. Some of them look at me in disbelief. I tell them that just when you think you have a handle on medicine, you too will meet someone like Jen.

REFERENCES AND FURTHER READING

Brotle C.D. *The role of mnemonic acronyms in clinical emergency medicine.* Toronto: University of Toronto; 2011.

Diem S.J., Lantos J.D., Tulsky J.A. Cardiopulmonary resuscitation on television: Miracles and misinformation. *N. Engl. J. Med.* 1996 June 13; *334*: 1578–82.

Harris D., Willoughby H. Resuscitation on television: Realistic or ridiculous? A quantitative observational analysis of the portrayal of cardiopulmonary resuscitation in television medical drama. *Resuscitation.* 2009; *80*: 1275–9.

Van den Bulck J.J. The impact of television fiction on public expectations of survival following inhospital cardiopulmonary resuscitation by medical professionals. *Eur. J. Emerg. Med.* 2002; *9*: 325–9.

STORIES IN MEDICAL EDUCATION AND TRAINING

Allan Cumming

Story: a narrative of incidents in their sequence.

Chambers Dictionary

For adult learners, learning experience needs to be orientated to life rather than to subject matter.

David et al., 1999

USING THE PATIENT'S STORY TO FOSTER LEARNING

The fundamental tenet of modern learning theory is that adults learn best when the subject matter is set in an appropriate context rather than presented in the abstract. For medical education, the most common context is the patient's story of a journey from health to illness and, hopefully, back again.

Some traditional medical curricula still require students to learn long lists of the names of muscles, or the minutiae of exotic biochemical pathways, without any explanation of how these relate to patient care. Opportunities to do this are routinely ignored. The Krebs cycle is presented without reference to the experience of patients with diabetic ketoacidosis. When students eventually meet such a patient and revisit their earlier learning, there is often a 'Eureka!' moment when the contribution of these invisible, intangible processes within the body to the patient's story suddenly becomes clear. Yet, with an integrated approach, this illumination, and the motivation and inspiration that it brings, could have been there from the start.

DOI: 10.1201/9781003409151-8

This realisation has led to the growth of what can be thought of as 'story-based learning' in medicine. Until the mid-1990s, this usually took the form of 'Clinical Correlation' sessions during the early years of the medical curriculum. For example, students who had spent many weeks being taught by pharmacologists about the names of drugs, their mechanisms of action, their pharmacokinetics and so on would be presented at the end of the module with a patient who was actually receiving one of the drugs for their clinical condition. The sessions were usually held in a lecture theatre, with an invited clinical doctor and a patient, in front of serried ranks of medical students. The patient would be asked to tell their story. Students would attempt to make connections between what they had been taught previously and the story that the patient recounted. The doctor running the session would try to facilitate this, but was not necessarily familiar with their prior learning. At worst, when the students were simply unable to 'join the dots', these sessions demoralised everyone concerned, and only emphasised the pre-clinical/clinical compartmentalisation which characterises traditional undergraduate curricula. At best – with a patient who told a relevant story well, an informed and prepared doctor who helped to elicit the significance of key points in the story and an engaged audience – they could inspire and encourage students, and remind them that the volume of context-free factual knowledge with which they had been presented had some relevance to their chosen vocation.

However, psychologists now consider that new learning is transferred most effectively into long-term memory by linking it with existing knowledge. This has led to a reversal of the order, with a switch from 'rule-example' to 'example-rule' teaching and learning. In the latter, the patient's story is the starting point for learning, and becomes the example (sometimes known as the 'trigger'). The rules (principles and factual knowledge) emerge from analysis of the story and are used to direct study. They can then be catalogued and cross-linked in the minds of learners in the context of that story.

PROBLEM-BASED LEARNING

In educational practice, various models of this type of teaching and learning exist. Problem-based learning (PBL) is the best known. It originated in McMaster University medical school, Hamilton, Ontario in 1969, spread to Europe via Maastricht University, Holland in the 1970s, and achieved widespread recognition and adoption worldwide from 1990 onwards. In addition to following the 'example-rule' principle, PBL gives students autonomy and responsibility to direct their own learning. They use elements in the story as signposts to relevant sources of information, and share that analysis and subsequent learning with other students in a small-group format. In 'classical' PBL tutorials, the facilitator is a process expert who is familiar with the story, but not necessarily a subject expert, and will ideally be a passive bystander, unless things go wrong. Box 8.1 presents a classical PBL trigger story.

BOX 8.1 A TALL GIRL

During the past few years, Ellen has grown tall very quickly. She has always been a fairly tall girl, but now at the age of 11, she stands head and shoulders above her peer group. People always take her to be older, which sometimes becomes wearisome. She wonders what will become of her. She still has not reached the age of puberty!

(David et al., 1999)

The signposts in this story are normal child growth; normal stages in secondary sexual characteristics; endocrine control of growth; psychological and social effects of abnormal height; and causes of, and treatments for, excessive growth.

Recently, new models of PBL have emerged that are not based on a single trigger story, but which require students to dissect the differences between multiple stories. Evidence suggests that this 'compare and contrast' task is even more effective in achieving transfer of knowledge into long-term memory.

OTHER MODELS OF STORY-BASED LEARNING AND ASSESSMENT

Other forms of story-based learning where the teacher may have a more active role include case-based learning (CBL), clinical case discussions and classic clinical bedside teaching. Indeed, the principle has become almost universally accepted in medical education; good lecturers will begin with a patient story even when teaching biomedical sciences, ethics or public health. The most recent trend in medical education is the 'flipped classroom', where students bring their (directed) prior learning to the lecture hall, and the 'lecture' then becomes an interactive discussion between the lecturer and their fellow students, exploring concepts and ideas in depth. Patient stories are often used as the basis for the advanced learning material, and lecturers can stretch the students by adding new elements to the story 'live'; for example, 'Ellen is now 16 and still has not had her first menstrual period'.

The progressive growth in the use of e-learning has fitted well with the trend towards story-based learning. Virtual patients, or even virtual families, can tell their stories online repeatedly at the learner's convenience. Computer-based algorithms can create 'branching' stories where the end of the story, or outcome, depends on choices made by the learner. This methodology can be used either for instruction or for assessment. An example of the latter (often called 'situational judgement tests') is given in Box 8.2.

BOX 8.2 A VIOLENT MAN

You are a single-handed GP in a remote rural practice. Mrs McInnes calls you to say that her husband has 'gone crazy again' and is smashing the furniture in their home. You go to the house. Mr McInnes, who is in his 60s and has a history of mental illness, is in a highly anxious, aggressive and disturbed state and is indeed destroying items of furniture. He has not harmed or threatened his wife or his children. Do you:

1. Phone the on-call psychiatrist at the district general hospital 30 miles away for advice?
2. Forcibly restrain him and sedate him with an injection of intramuscular chlorpromazine?
3. Call the police and ask them to arrest him?
4. Talk to him and try to calm him down?

If the candidate answers (2), the story ends with the death of the patient after a sudden fall in blood pressure.

The correct answer is (4).

(1) is a neutral response ('the psychiatrist makes some useful suggestions!').

(3) is incorrect. The patient has not yet committed any criminal act (the furniture is his own).

I encountered this question in an examination 30 years ago. The fact that I can recall every detail of the story, the underlying medical issues and correct responses demonstrates the power of medical storytelling in both learning and assessment.

This kind of story-based algorithmic approach has many similarities to narrative-based computer games, and similar techniques to those of computer gaming are being used increasingly to encourage immersion and engagement of the learner, provide positive feedback and make learning fun. It is an especially powerful tool in simulation teaching. Cardiopulmonary and trauma resuscitation and anaesthetic emergencies are particularly suited to this form of teaching. The new generations of manikins available are highly sophisticated, allowing many

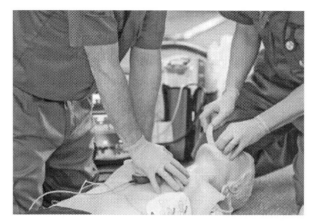

Figure 8.1 Simulation in medical training.

airway and surgical procedures to be performed with a high degree of realism and in real time. Given a trigger scenario – 'This patient has collapsed on the ward and is pulseless' – the actions of the operator, for example, in tracheal intubation, defibrillation, thoracostomy tube insertion, drug administration etc., can be overseen by the instructor and consequent changes in physiological parameters such as pulse rate, rhythm, blood pressure, respiratory effort etc., are relayed to the participant. The performance of a team, as well as an individual, can also be assessed, while the use of video allows post-scenario playback and focused discussion on the positive aspects of the case as well as errors and delays (Figure 8.1).

STORIES AND CONSTRUCTIVISM IN MEDICAL EDUCATION

Constructivism is currently the dominant theory in education and underpins the move towards a student-centred approach, peer tutoring and peer assessment. As originally defined by Jean Piaget in the 1960s, constructivism is 'a theory of knowledge that argues that humans generate knowledge and meaning from an interaction between their experiences and their ideas'. In the context of education, constructivism emphasises that individual learners construct meaning, taking into account their life experience, assumptions, motives, prior learning, the social context and language. The teacher teaches (or the patient tells their story), but the members of the class develop in their minds individual and different versions of what is said. In this process, teachers are facilitators rather than instructors. Learning is an active, social process. Students learn by sharing and comparing the principles, concepts and facts that they have accumulated from an educational experience, which in medicine is often an encounter with a patient and their story. In a real sense, each student, and indeed every doctor, creates their own version of every story, and learns from it.

BOX 8.3

A consultant physician, Dr F, was well known in his hospital as the 'go-to' person for difficult cases. Fellow consultants would routinely ask their team to refer to him patients in whom a diagnosis was not clear, since he would always provide a quick decision. However, junior doctors who worked with him soon realised that he always decided on the diagnosis on the basis of the information given over the phone by the referring doctor – usually a junior trainee. Rather than hearing the patient's story at first hand, Dr F would accept a second-hand version, and take his meaning from that. Very often he was correct.

On one occasion, a severely ill patient was transferred from another hospital with a provisional diagnostic label of systemic lupus erythematosus (SLE). The junior doctor on call referred him to the specialist by phone, giving a brief summary of the patient's condition and the possible diagnosis of SLE. The specialist looked at the patient's chest X-ray, stated that in his opinion the patient had SLE and recommended immediate, intensive immunosuppression therapy.

The junior doctor, who had reviewed the patient's records in detail and listened to his story in person, felt that it did not quite fit with a diagnosis of SLE and questioned the specialist on aspects of the story. However, by that time Dr F had 'nailed his colours to the mast', and the treatment went ahead.

The next morning the patient was much worse. Another specialist came, talked with and examined the patient in detail and made an alternative diagnosis of sub-acute bacterial endocarditis. This was confirmed with echocardiography and the patient had the infected valve removed.

The patient made a full recovery after several weeks of antibiotic therapy and the story had a happy ending.

The learning points of the story for the junior doctors were as follows.

- When making a clinical decision, always listen to the patient's story yourself, and beware of a 'given' diagnosis.
- Realise the dangers implicit in making snap decisions on the basis of incomplete information – but be aware that, in some situations, failure to decide may also have risks. Recognising those occasions is a key clinical skill.
- When colleagues create a story that conflicts with your own, listen to them and the patient, even if they are junior to you.

TEACHING STUDENTS TO HEAR THE PATIENT'S STORY

Teaching and assessing students' communication skills is a *sine qua non* of modern medical education. However, communication and history taking are not synonymous. The distinction can be blurred because in medical schools communication is usually taught and assessed in the context of a clinical encounter. Students may be superb communicators, but still lack the ability to hear and interpret a patient's story. Students must learn to give the patient space and time to tell their story and, most importantly, to actually hear what they say. They must recognise the crucial importance of timing and sequence – which often requires reiteration and clarification.

Patient management is increasingly protocol-driven, so students need to learn about pattern recognition and differentiation. The sifting of the rare condition from the common one is crucial. Is this patient's story one of deep venous thrombosis – or is it something similar but different? To use an ornithological analogy, the small brown bird in the tree outside your window is probably a sparrow – but it just might be an alpine accentor recently flown in from Switzerland!

To achieve this, the student must learn the importance of the contributions of synthesis, analysis and reflection. This means taking time to review the patient's story, link it with other relevant information, such as the results of investigations, and create a unified construct of the patient's situation. In turn this leads to clinical judgement and decision-making, a diagnostic formulation and a management plan. Students must learn about recording and onward transmission of the story – clinical hand-over skills, and accurate and comprehensive note-keeping, including the use of information technology.

The challenge for educators is to convey to students the endless fascination of hearing and interpreting the stories of patients, the 'Sherlock Holmes–like' persistence that is sometimes required to elicit the final clue in the tale, and the immense satisfaction when the pieces of the diagnostic jigsaw finally click into place. Examples, such as the one in Box 8.4, can help to illustrate this to students.

BOX 8.4

Mr W, a 50-year-old man, realises that he has not passed any urine for two days. Otherwise, he feels perfectly well. He goes to the local hospital for blood tests, which confirm that he has developed complete kidney failure. He is transferred to the specialist regional centre where dialysis is started. A junior doctor sits down to hear his story. After the standard questions, there is absolutely no clue pointing to any of the common causes of kidney failure. Various tests are done, but none indicates a possible cause. That evening the junior doctor returns to Mr W's bedside.

Junior doctor (JD)   Can you tell me again exactly what you have been doing in the last week or so?

Mr W   Well, we are building a new house. I have been working on it for the last couple of months.

JD   And what stage has it reached?

Mr W   Last week I was working on the bathrooms. We took delivery of two new baths, and I installed them.

JD   I see. What did that involve?

Mr W   The baths are delivered by the lorry driver in a protective plastic covering. I remove that, and then join them up to the pipes.

JD   How do you remove the plastic covering?

Mr W   Well, with a scrape. Sometimes it's stuck down, and I have to use a solvent to dissolve it and get it all off.

JD   What solvent did you use?

Mr W   Carbon tetrachloride [*JD gets very excited*]. But wait a minute, I know very well that carbon tetrachloride is toxic, so I take full precautions not to expose myself – rubber gloves, protective clothing, no spillage on my skin. Kept the windows open. So there is no way that I took any of it. [*JD now deflated.*]

JD   OK then. Can you just take me through in detail exactly how you set about doing this?

MrW   Once I've got most of the plastic off with the scraper, I carefully pour some of the solvent into the bath, leave it for a few minutes and then scrape the rest of it off. It takes about half an hour.

JD   [*This is the moment at which the light goes on.*] So, you are actually leaning over the bath to do the scraping?

Mr W   Yes, I actually have my head in the bath to get the right angle for scraping ...

JD   I'm sorry, I just need to Google something. Yes, I thought so. Carbon tetrachloride is volatile, the vapour is toxic and also it is heavier than air. The vapour would just have sat there in the bath while you stuck your head in. You would have been breathing it for half an hour ... [*Long silence!*]

Aspects of hearing a patient's story which impinge on medical ethics and professionalism include belief, cynicism, truth and falsehood. A fundamental precept of the doctor–patient relationship, which underpins the trust that patients place in doctors, is mutual truth and honesty. Yet every doctor has experienced situations where they know or suspect that the patient is either withholding part of their story, or fabricating it, for reasons which range from embarrassment to an intent to deceive. As a professional, the doctor must put that knowledge aside and not let it influence their interactions with the patient. Conversely, modern medical ethics emphasise the absolute imperative on the doctor to tell the patient 'the whole story', unless the patient themselves specifically asks them not to. Even in that situation, the decision to withhold information must be formally recorded, justified and revisited regularly.

We know from fiction that some stories are more affecting than others and draw the reader in emotionally. Were you in tears at the end? Many patients' stories are similarly deeply moving. Medical schools use 'empathy' as a marker of professionalism, and even look for evidence of it when selecting medical students. Clearly, it is a desirable attribute in a doctor. However, particularly early in their education and training, doctors can be drawn in to clinical situations in a way that is emotionally unsustainable and potentially damaging. Learning how to set boundaries on empathy and immersion is vital and often needs support from senior colleagues.

BOX 8.5 BOUNDARY SETTING

Anne is a middle-aged woman with liver disease. Her condition requires frequent blood samples and IV infusions. She is terrified of needles and finds these procedures very painful and distressing. Dr A is a junior doctor on the ward. He is very skilful at venous access and proud of his expertise. He finds the gratitude he receives from Anne when he is successful at the first attempt to be very emotionally rewarding, and shares in her distress when others are not successful. Eventually, Anne, with Dr A's tacit agreement, refuses to allow any other doctors or nurses to perform her venous access procedures. Even on his nights and weekends off, he comes to the hospital for this purpose. Increasingly, this extends to other aspects of her care – biopsies etc. A crisis comes when Dr A is unwell and unable to come to the hospital. At that point, a consultant intervenes. However, breaking the emotional bond between doctor and patient – and dealing with the practical implications – is deeply distressing for both parties.

THE LEARNER'S STORY

Every learner has their own story, and this has a major influence on their learning. Historically, universities and medical schools have failed to hear those stories. Students report that they feel anonymous and have no sense of 'belonging'. Often the university will know little or nothing about a student other than their performance in exams. These observations have led to the introduction of 'personal tutors' in many universities. These are academic staff who are required to meet regularly with students allocated to them, as individuals – even if the student is doing well. They do not just guide course choice, but help the student to regularly review and reflect on all aspects of their learning, including academic feedback, and to make action plans to reach their full potential. They aim to promote socialisation and engagement, and provide pastoral support when necessary. When the time comes to tell the story of the student's time at university, in the form of an employment reference, the personal tutor can give an accurate and informed account, in a way that was not possible before.

These concepts are being extended into the area of personalised, adaptive learning. Do all medical students need to follow courses of the same length? If a student can demonstrate the required learning outcomes after a shorter time, should they be allowed to do so? Or, if they have responsibilities like childcare or a need to work, should part-time study be available to them? Online learning can be blended with practical experiential learning in individualised study programmes that match the needs of each student and their story.

BOX 8.6

Ellie is a medical student from South-East Asia studying at a UK medical school. She is in Year 2 of the programme. Since starting at medical school, she has had few interactions with staff or with other students. She is quite shy, but the main issue is that, as a Muslim, she does not take alcohol. Every student event to which she might go seems to involve alcohol and intoxication. The social lives of other students seem to revolve around pubs and clubs. She spends her time studying in her room in the student residency. She is quite lonely and depressed but still gets good exam marks and the medical school views her progress as entirely satisfactory. Her parents back in Malaysia are happy because she is passing her exams.

At the start of Year 3 the university introduces a system of personal tutors. Her new personal tutor meets with her for an hour, and she is finally able to tell her story to someone who listens. The tutor invites her, along with the other ten students in her personal tutor group, to her house one evening for a meal. Soft drinks and beer in moderation are provided. Facilitated by the tutor, the group share their stories of life as medical students. The group includes another student in Year 4 of the course who has experienced similar problems, and talking to him is immensely helpful. The group agree to meet regularly for social events, taking their cultural and religious diversity into account. Ellie forms a study group with two of the other Year 3 students in the group; they work together in the library in the evenings with multiple breaks for coffee. Overall, the experience of Ellie at the medical school is transformed and she goes on to graduate with honours.

THE EDUCATOR'S STORY

Just as learners bring their own stories to their learning, medical educators bring their stories to their teaching. There is much current interest in the 'hidden curriculum', and the part played by role modelling, mentoring and 'osmotic' learning in helping students to develop as people and as medical professionals. Based on their story to date, educators will all have their own motivations and enthusiasms, which they are keen to impart to students. In many medical schools this energy is channelled to motivate students to undertake their own research projects working alongside investigators and their teams. Often, for the first time, the student gets an appreciation of what research truly involves, its frustrations, its excitements and the skill sets required.

The other side of this coin is that no educator is entirely free from some degree of bias and prejudice, be it conscious or unconscious. Traditionally, 'amateurs' – either clinicians or research scientists, without a specific training or vocation towards teaching – have conducted medical education. Increasingly, however, this has been recognised as unacceptable. New career paths have emerged for those with a particular interest and aptitude for medical education. In the UK, all doctors with an educational role are now required to undertake specific training for their education work. Such training helps educators to identify negative attitudes and behaviours that will affect their interaction with learners, as part of a long overdue professionalisation of medical education.

THE 'HAPPY ENDING' IN MEDICAL EDUCATION AND TRAINING

What is a good doctor and how do you make one? In 2002, an entire issue of the *BMJ* was devoted to this topic. The editorial concluded that they could not answer that question, and never could (Hurwitz & Vass, 2002). More recently, however, more positive approaches to this issue have emerged, based on the principles of outcome-based education (OBE). The UK General Medical Council (GMC), in its 2009 *Tomorrow's Doctors* statutory guidance to medical schools (GMC, 2009), says:

> *Graduates will make the care of patients their first concern, applying their knowledge and skills in a competent and ethical manner and using their ability to provide leadership and to analyse complex and uncertain situations.*

The council goes on to define in detail exactly what outcomes graduates must achieve during their time at medical school. They are categorised under the headings 'The doctor as scholar and scientist', 'The doctor as practitioner' and 'The doctor as professional'. Many other similar definitions of the outcomes of medical education now exist around the world – CanMEDS, Tuning (Medicine) and so on. So, rather unusually, in modern-day medical education we have a clear idea of how we want the story to end. Such an outcomes-based approach has the advantage that it does not stifle diversity in how medical schools design curricula and how learners approach their studies. Thus, many different stories in medical education can all reach the same conclusion.

The challenge to those who plan and organise medical education and training is to create stories which interest, motivate and involve the reader/learner; which make full use of new understandings of the process of learning; which can be told by expert staff with the time and energy to do it well; and which end with a competent and ethical doctor, fulfilled in their personal and professional life, delivering safe, effective patient care in whatever setting they choose to practise.

REFERENCES AND FURTHER READING

Cumming A., Ross M. The Tuning Project for Medicine: Learning outcomes for undergraduate medical education in Europe. *Med. Teach.* 2007; *29*: 636–41.

David T., Patel L., Burdett K., et al. *Problem-based learning in medicine: A practical guide for students and teachers.* London: RSM Press; 1999.

GMC. *Tomorrow's doctors: Outcomes and standards for undergraduate medical education.* GMC; 2009. Available at: www.gmc-uk.org/Tomorrow_s_Doctors_1214.pdf _48905759.pdf (accessed 24 May 2015).

Hurwitz B., Vass A. Editorial: What's a good doctor, and how can you make one? *BMJ.* 2002; *325*(7366): 667–8. www.royalcollege.ca/portal/page/portal/ rc/canmeds/canmeds2015.

A HOSPITAL'S STORY

Jim Huntley

Hospital – n. ME.

Hist. A house for the reception and entertainment of pilgrims, travellers, or strangers; any of the establishments of the Knights Hospitallers.

A charitable institution for the housing and maintenance of the needy; an asylum for the destitute, infirm, or the needy.

An institution or establishment providing medical or surgical treatment for the ill or wounded.

Adapted from *The New Shorter Oxford English Dictionary*, 1993

The whole earth is our hospital

Endowed by the ruined millionaire,

Wherein, if we do well, we shall

Die of the absolute paternal care

That will not leave us, but prevents us everywhere.

From T S Eliot, 'East Coker', 1943

This is a local story. On 10 June 2015, just shy of its 101st birthday, the Royal Hospital for Sick Children, Glasgow, 'Yorkhill' (Figure 9.1), is 'on the move' (NHS Greater Glasgow and Clyde, 2015a) to new premises in another part of the city. Much as I would like to believe in identity-teleportation for hospitals, in medicine and life, landscape

DOI: 10.1201/9781003409151-9

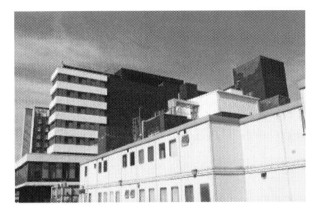

Figure 9.1 Royal Hospital for Sick Children, Yorkhill.

assumes a fundamental historical significance (Berger & Mohr, 1968). 'On the move' is a euphemism for 'dying', albeit with a corollary for a new institution to be born elsewhere: a phoenix rising from displaced ashes.

'Yorkhill' has been used and abused, and everywhere it bears the scars: stories of lives and loves, lived and lost. In the words of David Widgery, removed from their context: 'I'm watching something die and I wish I wasn't. Perhaps the best that can be done is to record the process' (Widgery, 1991).

Structure and function have been in decline for some time. The hospital was advanced in its 'final illness' when I came to work here, half a decade ago. The inside is similar to the outside – dirty and shabby – beaten up, scratched and defiled. Yorkhill stands in contrast to any number of hospitals, at home and abroad, where one cannot help but be impressed by the marble bleach-clean atria, the attention to showpiece aesthetics and light: pure, non-productive vacuous space. This latter is a halo effect (Dobelli, 2013), beauty subtending an aura of professionalism … that may be illusory. Despite the decay and incipient demise, I have felt more at home here in the hard-worked workshop than elsewhere in a frontispiece showroom.

Despite, or maybe because of, the near constant rain in Glasgow, the sign (Figure 9.2) at the bottom of the road is covered in grime. There is graffiti too. Past the sign is the 'hill' of Yorkhill, up and down which parents toil with buggies and wheelchairs, when the inadequate parking facilities are exhausted. On the rusting and paint-peeled right-hand fence is a sequence of yellow warning signs: 'Risk of death', perhaps relating to the power transformer on the other side. The pavement is cracked and resplendent with potholes, guaranteeing

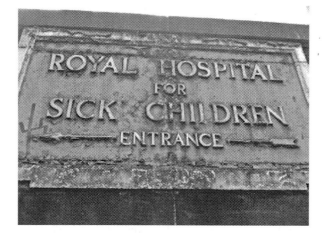

Figure 9.2 Main entrance sign.

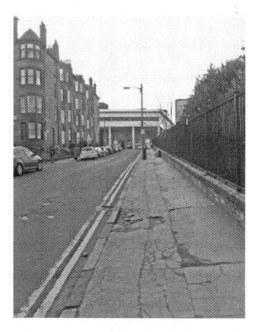

Figure 9.3 Yorkhill: the ascent to the Royal Hospital for Sick Children.

discomfort for buggy and wheelchair passengers and drivers alike (Figure 9.3).

Can we do no better than this? Consider Dr Norman Bethune, 80 years ago in circumstances of turmoil, in China, where at one of the base hospitals, the last stone step was missing. Bethune jumped the gap and asked the attendant if he minded jumping. The attendant replied that he did not. Bethune continued –

> *'And the convalescing patients – do* they *mind jumping?'*
> *The attendant's smile vanished. Together they brought a stone to replace the missing step. The incident went from mouth to mouth in the medical service with Bethune's moral: 'Never leave a stone unturned in caring for the wounded.'*

(Allan & Gordon, 1952)

In summer, the fence is suffused with florid green growth (Figure 9.4), which looks like Japanese knotweed (*Fallopia japonica*). Japanese knotweed won a prize at the 1886 Utrecht Flower Show, for being 'the most interesting newcomer' (Shaw & Tanner, 2008). Since then, its reputation has rather waned – it is now regarded as Britain's most pernicious weed (Shaw & Tanner, 2008). A Department for Environment, Food and Rural Affairs (DEFRA) study indicated it would cost upward of £1.5 billion to control it in Britain (Kurose et al., 2006). Unsurprisingly, its presence on a site adds substantial outlay to development costs. It has a powerful regenerative capacity from roots that may be 3 m deep and 7 m across, with shoots that can penetrate tarmac (Kurose et al., 2006), and its eradication is challenging. Like life's circumstances, *Fallopia japonica* can be vicious.

The road is one-way, except for a couple of consultant colleagues on their bicycles, looking for their dog-leg breaking sharp exit. It is strange that arrogance persists as a systematic complacency within

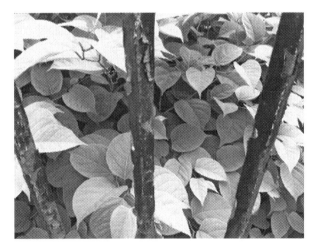

Figure 9.4 Fences and weeds: change and decay.

the hospital proper, whether this be doctors passing from patient to patient without washing their hands (as if bacteria might respect their eminence) (Daniels & Rees, 1999; Gawande, 2007), or disregarding the fundamentals of surgical protocol and discipline, moving through the main hospital in their theatre kit: hat, scrubs and clogs. We should stop flouting basic infection control measures, and, indeed, careering the wrong way down one-way streets.

Turning left, there is the walkway past the hospital outpatients. Here, the smokers congregate near the 'No Smoking' signs, by the open windows of the plaster room and the ventilation inlet to the cancer ward. Walt Whitman sits on my shoulder, cups his hand to my ear, and shouts: 'What good amid these, O me, O life?' (Whitman, 1892).

There are six lifts from the hall. At most, three function usefully. One is often set to go in the wrong direction, and two or three don't move, though the doors usually open and shut. On any given day, there is no obvious way to predict which lift has what properties. The management corridor is on the ground floor; if it were on the seventh, would the lifts have been fixed? Should you use the lifts? There is the option of the stairs (about which more shortly). This model of the 'Happy Vertical People Transporter' – as developed for the offices of *The Hitchhiker's Guide to the Galaxy* (Adams, 1980) – functions as a parody of a teenager's probability question and, as such, the hall is an antechamber, both physical and metaphysical, for what lies up or down. These lifts serve to tell us, though this was not their original function, that, in this building, whatever Einstein thought (Stent, 2006), God does indeed play dice.

I haven't the patience for a lift, so I use the stairs. These are of slippery stone, steep and of a step height just too much for young children. This would be fine except that they too have learnt not to play with the lifts, so they clamber up and down, and generally get under one's feet. The stairway barely admits two abreast, so people are usually stopping and starting; it is rare that you can get a decent run at it. The graces of this particular staircase are that it doesn't take up too much space, and that an object displaced centrally on the top floor will smash in the basement. It seems doubtful the designer consulted the fire department.

'Outpatients' score even higher. The consultation rooms seem like an adventure playground – but not because of a great collection of toys (there is no such collection). It is because of the traps – in a room here I count seven (but maybe I miss some): mouse-trap windows, scorching hot water, mouse-trap bins (×2), sharp-edged desks at eye-height for a three year old, door-stop (at most inconvenient place for a wheelchair user: 'get 'em on the rebound'), side-bars on the couch – sometimes helpful to prevent a fall, but another hinge-surprise danger-'toy'.

I obtained permission to take photographs within and around the hospital. I was excluded from photographing patients and the wards. In contrast, the NHS Greater Glasgow and Clyde booklet, *Celebrating a Proud History: The Royal Hospital for Sick Children 1882–2015* (NHS Greater Glasgow and Clyde Corporate Communications Team, 2015) is full of photographs of children, nurses and the wards. Historically, the wards look clean, spacious and light – optimistic even. There is little place for that outlook today. Over the last decade there has been a progressive erosion of nursing provision, numbers, in-hospital education and job security. Morale is low, despite the habitual strength, kindness and resilience of the nurses themselves. The wards are frenetic, the rush compounded by high bed occupancy and rates of turnover, or 'efficiency' on the managerial target sheet, as well as the need for real-time documentation.

The basement is no place for people, but it is a two-way shortcut, in and out (Figure 9.5). Here, among the failed cladding, the patched-up pipes, the furred-up stopcocks, amid the scars and fibrosis, the dust and cobwebs, there are 'signs of life': the abdominal sounds of the hospital. There is nutrition and excretion; fluid and gases are 'on the move'. The plumbing, be it hospital or human, starts perfect and slowly infarcts from the inside. There is nobility in this creaking hulking carcass. 'A hospital is like a battleship,' declared Sir Hector Cameron at the annual Yorkhill Hospital meeting in 1915. 'It is at its best when newly launched' (Robertson, 1972). Like so many ships from the Clyde, it has served its time. There are other escape exits, ways out, and into the light (Figure 9.6).

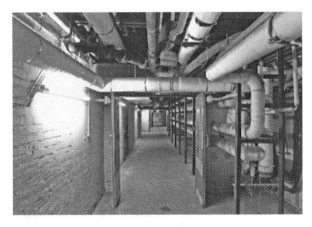

Figure 9.5 Royal Hospital for Sick Children: the bowels of the hospital.

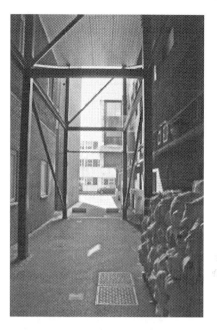

Figure 9.6 Side exit Royal Hospital for Sick Children: into the light.

Though I can hardly pretend it will change surgical outcomes, I will miss the view from the Theatre 5 window (Figure 9.7): the University of Glasgow, all that it represents in terms of the Scottish Enlightenment and key surgical and scientific figures; in front of it, statues of Lords Lister and Kelvin. Can I give the view a value? No – it does not appear on the 'Relative value unit' spreadsheet; it is an 'intangible'.

We recently had the fortune of a major upgrade to our electronic patient record and notes system. Unfortunately, this well-meant, top-down political directive has been instituted poorly and on an inadequate IT infrastructure. It has proven vulnerable to a 'never' event – crashing (Scottish Parliament, 2013) – and is disastrously slower and more vulnerable than the limited and part-paper system it replaced. Such problems, eminently predictable and predicted, seem unfortunately not to have been anticipated. Ominously, many such top-down initiatives devitalise the team and frontline ethos, whether this is in nursing wards, specialist departments or development of staff potentials.

Wouldn't any manager or director or leader or politician, who was managing (or directing or leading or politicking) by 'wandering around' (Peters & Waterman, 1982), notice something, be aware

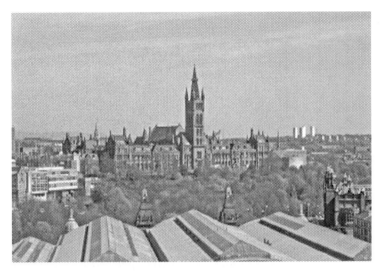

Figure 9.7 The view from Theatre 5: University of Glasgow.

and care, and go and make it right? Could it be that the reason for neglecting this myriad of problems is because they don't belong to an attributable target sheet? To our shame, Francis was right when he described 'a culture focused on doing the system's business – not that of the patients' (Francis, 2013).

There is little point in repairing the roof or the ventilation for the cardiac theatre as, on the other side of the river, the replacement hospital is almost built. Unsurprisingly, the new hospital has been touted as 'state-of-the-art' (NHS Greater Glasgow and Clyde, 2015b), and from further out as 'world-class' and 'gold standard' (BBC News, 2006). Let us hope so. What, or who, is going to make the new place work? Answer: the same team as has done of old. A friend uses the mnemonic 'POSSE' to describe the multidisciplinary team. It stands for 'Physiotherapist, Occupational therapist, Social worker, Speech therapist … and … Everyone else.'

I suspect that the POSSE – clinicians, nurses, physiotherapists, radiographers, technicians, orthotists, therapists, psychologists, play-leaders, secretaries, porters, social workers, receptionists, record managers and everyone else – will make it work, despite, not because of, the attention of politicians and executives. Yalof's book, *Life and Death: The Story of a Hospital* (Yalof, 1988), shows a sequence of sincere staff portraits – individual stories, motivations and beliefs – and how they combine to make the ethos of the hospital: the Columbia-Presbyterian Medical Center. Yalof has an optimistic introduction:

> *to know that it could stand up to close scrutiny, and that, warts and all,*
> *it would still emerge as the extraordinary place that it is.*

This fundamental co-operation is emphasised early:

> *'I'm a spoke in a wheel,' said the registrar in the Emergency Room, 'and*
> *if my co-workers and I are strong together, the wheel spins quickly and the*
> *patient's life is saved.'*

A hospital is nothing without its people. Perhaps the people are really its story. Contrast the vibrant Columbia-Presbyterian Medical Center with the bleak melancholy of the deserted United Community Hospital in Detroit, where poverty is reflected in the decaying abandoned buildings as well as the high infant mortality (Meyers & Hunt, 2014). Human geography recapitulates history.

The Glasgow children's hospital was founded in the district of Garnethill in 1882 ('Glasgow Hospital for Sick Children', 1882; Robertson, 1972; NHS Greater Glasgow and Clyde Corporate Communications Team, 2015). Prior to the inception of the NHS (1948), the children's hospital was a 'voluntary' hospital, answering what we perceive, with hindsight and from our privileged position in history, as a vicious need. A *Lancet* article of 1882 announced the opening and the need:

> *It is now well on for twenty years … since the appalling fact became*
> *known that of all the deaths in Glasgow upwards of 50 per cent were those*
> *of children under five years of age.*
>
> ('Glasgow Hospital for Sick Children', 1882)

The yearly mortality rate for the city was almost 3% of the population (NHS Greater Glasgow and Clyde Corporate Communications Team, 2015). The struggle to establish the hospital was in the face of vested interests, including obstructive political manoeuvring, particularly by the board of the Royal Infirmary and the Senate of the University of Glasgow (Robertson, 1972), to their shame.

The hospital moved to its current site in 1914, but after just over 50 years:

> *J J Burnet's building had reached the end of its days. Faults were found in*
> *the steel-and-concrete structure; the building was declared to be in a state*
> *of 'potential avalanche'.*
>
> (Robertson, 1972)

So it was demolished in 1966, rebuilt and reopened in 1971. In the best sense of the word, the hospital was founded, serially built and run on philanthropy ('love of humankind'). That culture continues today, albeit within the salaried NHS; the POSSE care, they lean on each other, depend on each other, far beyond the edges of sessional time commitments. A hospital is a complex system, by which I mean that its 'being' depends on a multitude of interactions between different agents (people in the POSSE) at the local level, independent of the chief executive. In short, there is no 'pace-maker'; the hospital should not be a strict hierarchy. The beauty of complex systems is in their emergent properties (real outcomes) that are of a different 'order' to the interactions between agents (Johnson, 2009). Robertson concludes her text, *The Yorkhill Story*:

> *Whatever dramas of paediatric progress may take place in the new hospital, it should never be forgotten that the Yorkhill story began with an ordinary dwelling house in Garnethill – and with a few men who had faith enough to fight for 20 years to establish a children's hospital in Glasgow.*

Similar praise is given by Chauncey Leake (1953) in his review of two books concerning hospitals, Manchester Royal Infirmary and Mount Sinai:

> *the biographies of institutions may be equally as interesting and important as the biographies of single individuals. Institutions, which are made up of changing groups of individuals, may often be successfully molded into agreeable and effective developments.*

Marshall Marinker (1998) has this to say, concerning the role of the hospital in health, diagnosis and disease:

> *The raison d'être of the modern hospital is the discovery and manifestation of diseases and their management. By definition it is in the hospital that the best diseases – the most florid, the most spectacular, the most intriguing – will manifest themselves.*

The hospital is a serious place, designed at some level for patients with serious problems. In his early work, 46 years ago, Crichton discussed an apparent conflict between doctor- and patient-centred hospital design:

> *The concept of a 'patient-orientated hospital' is fashionable at the moment ... People have recognised for a long time – at least twenty-five years*

– that hospitals are designed for the patient's needs only when those needs do not conflict with the doctors' convenience.

(Crichton, 1970)

An architect friend tells me: 'So many hospitals are designed like cow-pats.' Certainly, any number have an unremitting grimness, but I'm not sure that the fault lies solely with clinicians. Health professionals are concerned with maps and planning, patient flow, co-localisation of Emergency Departments with critical radiography etc. In his book, *Do No Harm*, the neurosurgeon Henry Marsh lays the blame for his specific instance with the Private Finance Initiative (PFI) (Marsh, 2014):

as with most PFI schemes the design of the building was dull and unorigi-nal. Nor was it cheap, since PFI has proved to be a very expensive way of building second-rate public buildings.

Hospitals must evolve with their society's economy and epidemiol-ogy. Marsh describes his struggle for the production of a roof garden, including years of campaigning and the raising of large charitable sums, culminating in 'the happy sight of the ward beds almost all empty' as patients and families alike moved out to enjoy the green space.

It is a small step in commentary from Crichton, concerning struc-ture, to narratives concerning function and attitude. Khadra pres-ages that keynote of the Francis report (Francis, 2013) – focusing on the system's business, not the patient's – by describing the hospital inpatient's perspective on nursing activities – the filling of forms and the 'writing in gigantic ledgers' (Khadra, 1999):

There are so many administrative layers now that it seems from where I lie in my hospital bed that the institution has been built to serve their needs and not mine.

(Khadra, 1999)

Cecil Helman also describes the inpatient's perspective:

Take what happens in hospitals, for example. For all their successes and technical wonders, the picture painted by many patients is often not a sym-pathetic one. They describe the hospital as a closed claustrophobic world, where – as in Oliver Sacks's A Leg to Stand On *[1991] – many undergo a process of depersonalisation, a loss of part of their identity. At a time of great anxiety, they find themselves away from family and friends, stripped of their usual clothing, dressed in a uniform of pyjamas or nightgown and lying as a numbered 'case' in a room filled with strangers. Soon other strangers in white coats will prod and question them, take away their blood and body fluids for analysis, while huge whirring machines will point at, or probe, one part of their body after another.*

(Helman, 2003)

Sacks's brilliant little book is often held to give an account of an unthinking and unsympathetic surgeon, as well as Sacks's own depersonalisation. However, there is much that is positive about clinicians and health professionals. In particular, early in his travails, after his accident, Sacks (1991) describes a young Norwegian surgeon who

remains most vividly and affectionately in my mind, because in his own person he stood for health, valour, humour – and a most wonderful, active empathy for patients ... He leapt and danced and showed me his wounds, showing me at the same time his perfect recovery.

Elsewhere, Helman (2006) maintains:

hospitals have become factories, yet another form of industrial mass-production in our society, with the raw material of sick people being fed in at one end, and healthy people being produced en masse at the other. Or at least, that's the aim. But they turn us from people into products at a very crucial time in our lives, a time of anxiety and ambiguity, where the very threads that hold our sense of personhood together are in danger of being torn apart. Many hospitals have become businesses, dedicated solely to production – if not to profit, to cost effectiveness – but without considering the other types of cost that result from this approach: social, emotional, spiritual. They have become businesses run by managers, primarily for the benefit of other managers, accountants and of other executives higher up in the food chain. No wonder so many patients are unhappy with hospitals these days.

Bynum (2008) notes:

Despite the problems, hospitals are here to stay. They have three particular features that make them indispensable: sophisticated diagnosis, acute care, and surgery.

The sentiments of Helman, Sacks, Khadra and Crichton need to be taken as a challenge: within the context of limited resources and utilitarian ethics (the greatest good by the greatest number) to 'retain humanity'. They also need to be contrasted with the grass-roots fury often expressed at the prospects of local hospital closure. Hospital history, ethos, leadership, design and art all present important challenges that must be met by greater initiative than a trite and banal mission statement.

This fragment of one hospital's story is not unusual. Similar stories surely relate to many, worldwide. A building, an inanimate collection of bricks and concrete enclosing a convoluted, dysfunctional organisation has its own intrinsic narrative. Its story is as valid as ours and those of our patients. I advance the idea, as this flawed, imperfect complex hospital dies, that it has represented the highest form of human and societal endeavour. In her 'Afterword', Yalof (1988) parallels hospital and humankind, as she predicts:

> *One more thing I am sure of: Things will still be moving along. In this sense, the heart of a hospital emulates and even outdoes the human heart. It keeps right on beating.*

The hospital is a concerted philanthropic endeavour, perhaps defining of 'civilisation'. It is both a metaphor and a yardstick of the best that humankind can offer: not as good as we might aspire to, but so much better than our worst behaviour. It is a global story.

POSTSCRIPT FOR THE SECOND EDITION

Evening of 17 May 2022. Seven years 'since closure'; there are signs of life – at the main entrance there has been a limited rechristening: 'West Glasgow Ambulatory Care Hospital', but I see no one, and the car parks are empty. Appendages of the hospital have been lopped off (interconnecting bridge corridors and the like); the advisory 'signs' are dirty and missing letters. I am reminded of Richard Selzer's story 'Mercy' (Selzer, 1980) in which the doctor tries to alleviate a patient's pain with an excessive dose of opiate, to 'put him out of his misery', but he fails. No one has had the decency to quite finish off Yorkhill either.

REFERENCES AND FURTHER READING

Adams D.N. *The restaurant at the end of the universe.* London: Pan; 1980.

Allan T., Gordon S. Chapter 50. In: *The scalpel, the sword: The story of Doctor Norman Bethune.* Toronto: McClelland & Stewart; 1952.

BBC News. *Site for £100m hospital announced.* 14 March 2006. Available at: http://news.bbc.co.uk/1/hi/scotland/4804778.stm (accessed 4 June 2015).

Berger J., Mohr J. *A fortunate man: The story of a country doctor.* Readers Union edition. London: Penguin Press; 1968.

Bynum W. Medicine in the modern world. In: *The history of medicine: A very short introduction.* Oxford: Oxford University Press; 2008.

Crichton M. *Five patients*. New York: Alfred Knopf; 1970.

Daniels I.R., Rees B.I. Handwashing: Simple, but effective. *Ann. R. Coll. Surg. Engl.* 1999; *81*: 117–18.

Dobelli R. Everyone is beautiful at the top: Halo effect. In: *The art of thinking clearly*. London: Hodder & Stoughton; 2013.

Francis R. *Public inquiry: Report of the Mid Staffordshire NHS Foundation Trust public inquiry*. Vol. 1. *Analysis of evidence and lessons learned (part 1)*. London: The Stationery Office; 2013. Available at: www.midstaffspublicinquiry.com/sites/default/files/report/Volume%201.pdf (accessed 3 April 2013).

Gawande A. On washing hands. In: *Better: A surgeon's notes on performance*. London: Profile Books; 2007.

Glasgow Hospital for Sick Children. *Lancet*. 1882; *1*: 1053.

Helman C. Introduction: The healing bond. In: Helman C., ed. *Doctors and patients: An anthology*. Oxford: Radcliffe Medical Press; 2003.

Helman C. Hospital. In: *Suburban Shaman: Tales from medicine's frontline*. London: Hammersmith Press; 2006.

Johnson N.F. Section 1.4 The key components of complexity. In: *Simply complexity: A clear guide to complexity theory*. Oxford: Oneworld; 2009.

Khadra M. What cost, compassion? In: Slater S., Downie R., Gordon G. et al., eds. *The magic bullet and other medical stories*. Glasgow: Royal College of Physicians and Surgeons of Glasgow; 1999.

Kurose D., Renals T., Shaw R., et al. *Fallopia japonica*, an increasingly intractable weed problem in the UK: Can fungi help cut through this Gordian knot? *Mycologist*. 2006; *20*: 126–9.

Leake C.D. Portrait of a hospital, 1752–1948, to commemorate the bi-centenary of the royal infirmary, Manchester. *Yale J. Biol. Med.* 1953; *25*: 289–90.

Marinker M. Sirens, stray dogs, and the narrative of Hilda Thomson. In: Greenhalgh T., Hurwitz B., eds. *Narrative based medicine: Dialogue and discourse in clinical practice*. London: BMJ Books; 1998.

Marsh H. Oligodendroglioma. In: *Do no harm: Stories of life, death, and brain surgery*. London: Weidenfeld & Nicolson; 2014.

Meyers T., Hunt N.R. The art of medicine. The other global South. *Lancet*. 2014; *384*: 1921–2.

NHS Greater Glasgow and Clyde. New South Glasgow Hospitals. *NSGH on the move … Issue 4*. Glasgow: NHS Greater Glasgow and Clyde; 2015a.

NHS Greater Glasgow and Clyde. *New children's hospital*. Glasgow: NHS Greater Glasgow and Clyde; 2015b.

NHS Greater Glasgow and Clyde Corporate Communications Team. *Celebrating a proud history: The Royal Hospital for sick children, 1882–2015*. Glasgow: NHS Greater Glasgow and Clyde; 2015.

Peters T.J., Waterman R.H. Jr. Hands on, value-driven. In: *In search of excellence*. London: HarperCollins; 1982.

Robertson E. *The Yorkhill story: History of the Royal Hospital for sick children, Glasgow*. Glasgow: Yorkhill and Associated Hospitals Board of Management; 1972.

Sacks O. *A leg to stand on*. London: Picador; 1991.

Scottish Parliament. *Official report: Meeting of the Parliament; Wednesday, 2 October 2013*.

Selzer R. Mercy. *The Iowa review.* 1980; 11: 117–9.

Session 4: 23167–23172. Edinburgh: APS Group Scotland. Available at: www
.scottish.parliament.uk/parliamentarybusiness/report.aspx?r=9030&mode=pdf
(accessed 6 June 2015).

Shaw R., Tanner R. Weed like to see less of them. *Biologist.* 2008; *55*: 208–14.

Stent G.S. Francis Crick. *Proc. Am. Philosoph. Soc.* 2006; *150*: 467–74.

Whitman W. O me! O life! In: *Leaves of grass.* Philadelphia, PA: David Mackay;
1892.

Widgery D. On yer bus. In: *Some lives! A GP's East end.* London: Sinclair-
Stevenson; 1991.

Yalof I. *Life and death: The story of a hospital.* New York: Random House; 1988.

A PARAMEDIC'S STORY

Joel Symonds

I'm called on a late summer evening to a man in his 20s who has been knocked off his bike. The evening is bright, but cooling – summer has taken its temperature home a few weeks early, but the light in the late afternoons still holds empty promises of picnics and drinks in the park, of late gentle walks home in the sunshine, or lazily enjoying an ice cream with a bag of wet, sandy clothes. The promises are empty; the light is there, the warmth has gone.

A man has been knocked from his bike. Those facts are true. A man was on his bike, and now he is not. But this factual and innocuous description does nothing to illustrate the full picture.

I pull up to find two ambulance crews resuscitating him in the road.

He is a man … but only just. His stubble is there, but soft and blond. His shoulders are broad, but the rest is adolescent, as though his skeleton bought his frame on sale and is waiting for him to grow into it.

Age is difficult, but we guess at 20; his fake ID says 19, the police know him as 15.

The poppers on his tracksuit bottoms have ripped away at the ankle, one gaudy, blood-slicked trainer lies in the gutter. This is no working man commuting home from the office. This is a kid riding a bike after tea.

A car nearby has lost a wing, a mirror, its windscreen crystalline. The driver is another young man, though with maybe five years on the child in the road. He reels wildly between the police, the patient and a phone call to a recovery service and body shop.

The ambulance crew welcome me and as a team we communicate in checklists, algorithms and mnemonics. We systemise, categorise,

DOI: 10.1201/9781003409151-10

objectivise. We devise, deduce and measure. In the face of sudden, catastrophic chaos, we calculate and numerate in an attempt to gain control of the desperate human tragedy that is unravelling within the circle of our fluorescent shoulders.

Dusk falls.

I run my hands across the rhythmic railings of his chest; his belly is so thin I can feel individual organs. His hips are angled and twisted with an asymmetry that neither evolution nor creator ever intended. His legs are long and lithe, the sort that you can only achieve by playing endless hours of football in the park with friends because you have no other responsibilities. I slide my hands across his scalp and feel rocky lumps and shards of skull crunching beneath my fingers. His hair sticks to my hands when I pull them away, like I'm an over-tousling uncle who plays too rough.

The algorithm demands action and sacrifice, it calls for exploration, probing and drainage.

I draw a scalpel along the skin between his ribs, punch forceps through his chest wall and push my fingers inside. Waves of blood retch from the holes I've cut and the hot, wet edge of his lung nudges against my fingertips like an old blind dog. His skull is shattered, his chest awash and drowning in blood in all the wrong places.

He's done. We stop. An officer is dispatched to his house to tell his mum and dad.

We tuck him under an icy white blanket and leave him in the road. A priest emerges from one of the nearby houses, lights a candle and asks if I'd be offended if he prays.

He lies ten feet from my bumper; when I sit in the driver's seat my headlights automatically click on and illuminate him. The tarmac is blacker than black, his arms stretched out, cruciform. I can see a long stripe of him where the blanket doesn't quite meet the road. His neck, shoulders, flanks and legs, pasty and polar white, are growing paler and bluer by the second as blood settles in his abandoned circulation. Just under his armpit, the ragged, dark red slash from my scalpel is lurid and obscene.

The streetlights come on, signalling to us all that it's time to go home, where our mums and dads are waiting.

I think about his mum.

I think about this woman sitting in an anonymous armchair somewhere, elsewhere in town. Not yet fretting since she doesn't yet know he's late.

I think of this woman who bore him and birthed him, unmarked and unblemished. This woman who gazed on every square inch of his perfect skin, who saw the yawning, waiting potential of his unwritten story. This boy with skin the colour of cream, this blank bolt of linen, this sheet ready for an epic opus to be recorded across its space.

His skin became a log, a manuscript. He lived and wrote his story upon its surface with the help of those around him. In tally marks, scrapes and scars his skin recorded capers and misadventures, near misses and family legend.

For those first few months she was editor-in-chief, she knew every milk-spot and pimple, every rash and flush of heat. When he was 18 months old, she found him, one morning, his pyjamas stained with blood. He'd mindlessly raked the top from a bug bite in his sleep, showing her in scarlet splotches that he held new autonomy on the story that was to be told. As a rambunctious toddler, his shins and knees bloomed in impressionist purples and blues from more bumps and bangs than she could track.

She wasn't alone, others rushed and lobbied to keep her as primary author; one day she collected him from school with a plaster on his knee. His teacher had filled out an incident form, had validated and enumerated, logged and catalogued. They passed this note to his mum as editor-in-chief, ensuring she was fully abreast of every clause as it was written.

At nine years old he slipped on the beach; she saw his milky white skin vanish suddenly behind Grecian rocks on a packaged seaside. He ran to her, weeping, blood and sand and tears smearing on his face, his eyebrow split into a gurning grin. Years later they tell the story of the kindly local doctor, the tapas restaurant that stayed open late for them, how his Dad carried him back to the villa, how they weren't sure if he was concussed, or had just had too much ice cream. His scar became family lore.

At 12, he'd vomited all night, moaning and grasping his tummy – they had ended up in A&E at three in the morning and by breakfast time (not that he was allowed any) they'd wheeled him into theatre for his appendix. She's brave when she tells this story, but to her closest friends she's tearily recounted how small he looked on the hospital trolley. The laparoscopic constellation of scars across his belly is barely visible.

There is space upon his skin for so many other stories, were it not for tonight's events.

At 19, he lost a bet and found himself in a grubby Magaluf tattoo parlour, his friends braying at the window, consumed with admiration, relief, lager and fear for what his mum would say.

At 36, his wedding ring would snag on a motor's errant flywheel, tugging at the hand as the gold held tight, for better or for worse. The skin stripped off like fruit peel as the ring came away; they'd darn him back together like a woollen glove. He'd wear the ring on a chain afterwards.

At 84, the council will have stopped sweeping the wet leaves off the path outside; he would only be going out for a paper. They'd unzip his hip and slot in a pin. He'd be in for a week, cared for by nurses too young to understand his jokes about the bionic man.

But these stories will remain unwritten; they are drafts that never made the final cut.

He has come to us alone, an Icarus with scrappy, fledgling feathers; his skin not quite his own as he stretches and spins at the very limits of parental orbit, the centrifugal force of his desperation to grow up dashing him, and his cheap fake ID, against the rocks of adulthood. Here in the darkness, emptying into the road around us, he has found a terrible new co-author in me. I am a stranger with no knowledge of his hopes and plans, his aspirations or fears. I have no understanding of the family narrative I am leaving on the cutting-room floor, what devastation the removal of his story will bring. I am an interloper in his script; I emerge from the wings, a hitherto unknown character to neatly bring the story to a close. Deus ex machina in surgical gloves.

Like some blundering imperial archaeologist, I have smashed and cut away at the most central parts of him, raking around in the breathless mausoleum of his ribs. More butcher than surgeon, I have seen and touched parts of him that his mum, who once knew his every inch, will never see or know. Nor should she. No mother should feel her son's pleura against her knuckles, his lungs lapping at her fingers. Far better for those experiences to be recorded as hospital notes, the medic's bizarre, anonymous intimacy removed from his story and instead categorised, organised and archived somewhere safe where no one has to read it out loud.

His story ends. He becomes a case, a reflection, a cautionary tale to students.

His story becomes just a chapter in *mine*.

YOU SHOULD WRITE

Jim Huntley

Man is superior to the higher apes not only in opposing his thumbs but also in the using of symbols, mostly spoken or written words, to convey his meaning.

R A J Asher, 1943

Observe, record, tabulate, communicate. Use your five senses. Learn to see, learn to hear, learn to feel, learn to smell, and know that by practice alone you can become expert.

Sir William Osler, *The Quotable Osler*, 2003

The question, O me! So sad, recurring – What good amid these, O me, O life?

Answer

That you are here – that life exists and identity,

That the powerful play goes on, and you may contribute a verse.

Walt Whitman, 1892

Clinic is running late. The boy has diplegic cerebral palsy, and has had previous well-meant orthopaedic operations. Unfortunately, these surgeries were devoid of any understanding of the sequelae of over-lengthening biarticular muscles. Now, with growth, he has subsided into severe crouch: sagittal Z-collapse, 'gone off his legs', with all that entails for future dependence. This is iatrogenic harm (our words, like our Medicine, from the Greek roots: 'iatros' – physician, 'gen' – caused). For the last year, he has been unable to pivot transfer, so he

DOI: 10.1201/9781003409151-11

depends on his parents to lift him. They are devoted. In the future he will put on weight; as they get older, they will weaken, and life will be tough, the burden heavier. We talk, and I ask him about school, and my 'unscripted' question about his favourite subject. It transpires that it is English, or more precisely: writing.

His father tells me proudly: 'He writes so so much, Doctor, and the little pieces he lets us see are brilliant.'

I examine him, supine and prone, filling in my proforma for passive range, every direction, every lower limb joint, assessment of selectivity, lags, power, spasticity, rotational profile, and 'special tests'. Afterwards with him re-dressed and lifted to his wheelchair, with the X-rays on the screen, we talk. Or rather I talk. I give a variation of my standard script: I tell the family what multi-level surgery involves, and the rationale and the aims of doing so many operations on one day, and running an epidural for three days afterwards, and the intensive rehabilitation over two years.

He looks at me and starts to sob, great racking sobs. His parents hug him, one from either side, and sit quietly, waiting for him to talk, but he cries for a long time and then the tears ebb, and he sits staring into space.

★★★

This chapter was going to be straightforward, with clear headings and a structure, like a medical clerking or a scientific paper. I had a clear map, starting at the beginning and running linearly to the end. But the point is that writing is not just an exposition; rather, it's an exploration. The journey and the thinking curl back on themselves and wander off in unanticipated directions. Thoughts extend.

Why write? I have collected a number of articles (e.g., Fogarty, 2013; Stein, 2013) and books on writing, 'How to' and 'Why to'. I recognise my selection bias. I already want to write. I read them to self-justify. Maybe some will help. Like so many texts, they reach to the choir, to the already converted. I want to talk beyond the choir … maybe to you.

George Orwell discusses the writer's motives in terms of early development, framing their influences in terms of particular time and environment, in a kind of amateur, self-evident relativism. He suggests that, aside from the need to earn a living (a dubious method), there are four great motives: (1) sheer egoism, (2) aesthetic enthusiasm, (3) historical impulse ('a desire to see things as they are') and (4) a political purpose … 'a desire to push the world in a particular direction' (Orwell, 1994). All seem to be more general motivations for doing anything: sport, acting … even medicine … we are hardly short of our monstrous egoists, our aesthetic possibilities, an arcane history of ideas and biases, and as for politics (potentially overlapping with sheer egoism), if the trajectory of a medical/surgical career is decline, there are always administration, safeguarding, meetings, important committees to be sat on, and 'the College'.

Margaret Atwood addresses the question of motive, in the 'words of writers themselves' (Atwood, 2003a): 'to record … set down … excavate … satisfy … express … create … hold a mirror … justify … Graphomania … logorrhea … serve … subvert … experiment … speak … praise'. She compounds her purposeful failure 'on the subject of motives' with authoritative wit, not least of Samuel Beckett: 'writing was all he was good for'. She concludes her introduction to *On Writers and Writing* with a quote from a medical student from 40 years before, concerning the inside of the human body: 'It's dark in there'. She believes that writing has to do with entering darkness and bringing something back into the light.

In 'Aren't I Lucky? I Can Write!' Richard Asher avows an unenthusiastic attitude. The process of writing is 'so laborious and tedious that authors often despair of getting their ideas on to paper at all'; although admitting that he can write, he professes: 'I am not particularly proud of it, nor do I get a great deal of pleasure from it'. He emphasises the disproportionate amount of time spent revising and re-revising text, with every revision a laboured improvement. He concludes that writing is done 'more by toil than by gift. Is it worth it? I really don't think it is. Then why do I write? Honestly I don't know' (Asher, 2015a).

Sir William Osler (1849–1919), regarded by many as the father of modern medical education and practice, believed that physicians should 'always note and record the unusual … Publish it. Place it on permanent record as a short concise note. Such communications are always of value' (Osler 2003; Caban-Martinez & Garcia Beltran, 2012). Additionally, he advocated for the humanities:

> *Nothing will sustain you more potently than the power to recognise in your humdrum routine, as perhaps it may be thought, the true poetry of life – the poetry of the commonplace, of the plain, toil-worn woman, with their loves and their joys, their sorrows and their griefs.*

Believing that a physician should be taught a combination of science and humanities, it is a small step to invoke his support for humanistic short-form writing.

'The Bell Curve' (Gawande, 2004) is an essay about geographic mortality variations for cystic fibrosis. I give copies of this piece to most of my fellows in training, for their reflections. It is about variation in standards of care, about attitudes and actions that make a differ-ence, about what it takes to be a genuine positive outlier or positive deviant. On one hand, we should aspire to the highest standards. On the other, it can be difficult to work in teams with demanding maver-icks. Positive deviance is an 'approach … to change … [by] … people whose uncommon but successful behaviors or strategies enable them to find better solutions … despite facing similar challenges and having no extra resources' (Berkowitz & McCarthy, 2013; cited in Beaulieu, 2013). Gawande also gives five suggestions on how to be a positive deviant in Medicine (Gawande, 2007; Beaulieu 2013):

- Do not complain
- Be an early adopter (change!)
- Ask an unscripted question
- Count something
- *Write something*

To these I would add:

- Read more (Descartes on reading 'To converse with those of other centuries is almost the same as travelling' [Adair, 2007])
- Engage with the visual arts

So, again, why write? Asher doesn't know but knows he doesn't know. Orwell thinks he knows but doesn't. Atwood knows but won't tell us. Osler knows what is best for us. Gawande wants to be a posi-tive deviant.

Paul Graham in a short essay, 'Writing, Briefly' says that 'Writing doesn't just communicate ideas; it generates them' and extends the message that, if you don't write, 'You'll miss out on most of the ideas writing would have generated … expect 80% of the ideas in an essay to happen after you start writing it, and 50% of those you start with to be wrong' (Graham, 2005).

Although there are simple practical strategies for 'practicing narrative-based medicine' directly at the level of patient encounters (Peterkin, 2012), here we confine ourselves to writing, and particu-larly writing short-form 'story', and implicitly in 55-word chunks. There are few true confines; music arises from an octave of only eight notes. This chapter is more than mere encouragement and tangential reflection. It is an exhortation to write, not merely for expression, but for thought extension and crystallisation.

Thinking about volition, maybe it is useful to consider its apathetic obverse, 'not writing' in 55 words.

BOX 11.1 WHY I DON'T WRITE

Nothing to say, no reason to articulate thought,
Nor extend it. Why climb? Is there a summit?
The mist is thick – nothing to see, and
Climbing is dangerous. For the view, they would
Fold the picture away, in a coffin, or burn it.
The past is irrelevant.
The present is dead.
The future is nought.

Again, Paul Graham: 'If writing down your ideas always makes them more precise and more complete, then no one who hasn't written about a topic has fully formed ideas about it. And someone who never writes has no fully formed ideas about anything nontrivial' (Graham, 2022), and Atwood (2003b):

> tell, if not a story, at least a mini-story … the crooked is made straight, or, the age being what it is, possibly more crooked; at any rate there's a path. There's a beginning, there's an end, not necessarily in that order … events take place, in relation to other events. That's what time is … one damn thing after another, and the important word in that sentence is *after*.

We will come back to time, later.

Nowadays we rarely repay the debts we owe our best teachers. Medicine is a teaching profession and in the times of the Hippocratic oath, physician's mentors were honoured and revered (Antoniou et al., 2010):

> To hold him who taught me this art equally dear to me as my parents, to be a partner in life with him, and to fulfill his needs when required; to look upon his offspring as equals to my own siblings, and to teach them this art, if they shall wish to learn it, without fee or contract; and that by the set rules, lectures, and every other mode of instruction, I will impart a knowledge of the art to my own sons, and those of my teachers, and to students bound by this contract and having sworn this Oath to the law of medicine, but to no others.

> (Hulkower, 2016)

The commitment to teaching (but not to teachers) remains, albeit watered-down, in modern abridged versions. For instance, in the Edinburgh Medical Oath (Green, 2017):

'I will constantly seek to gain in knowledge and understanding, and to pass on the art and science of medicine to others, as my teachers have done before me.' Despite, or maybe because of, the erosion of respect for our teachers, for our history, it seems right to make the Hippocratic pilgrimage, back to our origins, to breathe the air of our ancestors, to tread where they trod, to see the view our teachers' teachers saw, to stand on the top level of the Asklepion of Kos (Figure 11.1).

John McPhee (McPhee, 2017), considers the difficulties of structure in long-form nonfiction, and invokes a lesson from Olive McKee, his English Teacher from Princeton High: 'each composition had to be accompanied by a structural outline, which she told us to do first … the idea was to build some form of blueprint before working it out in sentences and paragraphs.' There is a fundamental point here: the alliance of the visual with the textual. As previously (Huntley, 2004) paraphrased from John Berger's *Ways of Seeing* (Berger, 1972): 'images subsist at a more fundamental level than words'. We will come to images, to pictures as prompts, as 'ways in'. Here, we are going to be concerned with short-form, and so short a short-form (55 words) that structure can be imposed somewhat on the hoof.

Paradoxically it seems there are more forms of 'short-form' than 'long-form'. Some have achieved a certain salience: short columns (Holub, 1992), fillers, vignettes, epigrams (Moran, 2018), aphorisms (Moran, 2018), anecdotes, fables, drabbles (exactly 100 words) (Monty

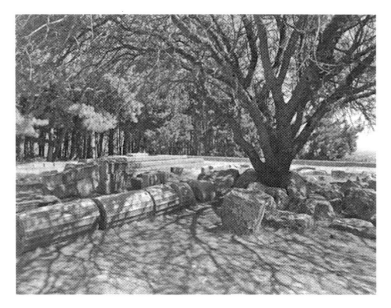

Figure 11.1 Top level of the Asklepion of Kos.

Python, 1971), 55-word stories (Moss, 1995; Grant, 2008; Fogarty, 2010; Childress, 2017; Fogarty et al., 2013; Laverty et al., 2017), and Grooks (Hicks, 1966; Hein, 2002).

Miroslav Holub, immunologist and man of letters, gave a list of rules for writing short columns (Holub, 1992), emphasising: (i) 'light disposition', (ii) 'certain facetiousness', (iii) 'mundane topic', (iv) 'if more demanding … must draw explicitly on personal experience', (v) 'fruit of physiological satiety'. He finally points up the freedom of short-form from rules by dispelling all such nonsense in his last line: 'It bothers me a lot that I haven't followed them more closely.'

Before coming to the promised 55-word story, I digress again, this time into the story of the 'grook', which is really the story of the power of a very few words as a form of action. Piet Hein, the Danish polymath, was the inventor of the polycube puzzle Soma and the game Hex, identifier of the 'super-ellipse' and, despite being 'trapped within a minor language' (Hicks, 1966), the originator of 'grooks' (a grook is a short epigrammatic text, usually poetic, often whimsical) (Gardner, 2013). Grooks are now published worldwide, but were originally for the Danish newspaper *Politiken* at the time of Nazi occupation. Hein was president of the Anti-Nazi Union when Germany invaded Denmark – as he said:

> *That was not the best thing to be on April 9, 1940. I had to go underground. It was a strain not being able to say anything. Then I found a way, those small poems, I grasped the word grook out of empty air … I believed that there would only be four or five grooks in all. Had I known there would be 7,000 I would have taken more care what I called them.*
>
> (Hicks, 1966)

These grooks were encoded messages of resistance, resilience and anti-collaboration for Danish readers. Box 11.2 provides an example, in just 25 words.

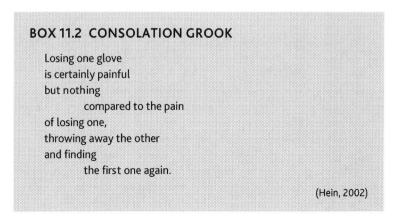

BOX 11.2 CONSOLATION GROOK

Losing one glove
is certainly painful
but nothing
    compared to the pain
of losing one,
throwing away the other
and finding
    the first one again.

(Hein, 2002)

The 55-word story originated with Steve Moss in 1987, when he challenged readers of the *New Times* to develop a 'lean story' in 55 words or less. The best were collated in *The World's Shortest Stories* (Moss, 1995). Moran emphasises the primacy of the sentence in writing: 'a sentence is not about self-expression but about editing your thoughts into a partly feigned fluency, building a ladder of words up to a better self'; and elsewhere: 'in writing, meaning derives from just four things: syntax, word choice, punctuation and typography' (Moran, 2018). With only 55 words, there is little space for many sentences, so attention to their structure must be immaculate, to herald a self-contained bubble of thought, nevertheless with sufficient scope for ambition and invention. The 55-word format has been appropriated by Medicine and explored in seminars (Fogarty, 2010), courses (Childress, 2017) and collections (Scheetz & Fry, 2000; Christianson, 2002; Grant, 2008; Fogarty et al., 2013; Laverty et al., 2017). 'Storying early, storying often, in 55 words or more, physicians can hold to humanistic and ethical understandings of patient care and of themselves' (Childress 2017). Childress further notes: 'Perhaps most importantly, anyone can write a 55-word story'.

So that means YOU!

Fogarty produced guidelines for writing such 'small jewels', that I have modified in Table 11.1. Though the rules are few, she suggests that good 55-word pieces include 'the key elements of narrative':

(1) Setting (When and Where?)
(2) Character(s) (Who?)
(3) Conflict (something has to happen!) (What and How?)
(4) Resolution (Why?)

Richard Asher borrowed Kipling's 'six wise men and true' for medical writers (Asher, 2015b).

> *Their names are what, and why, and when,*
> *And how, and where, and who.*

He suggests that 'most scientific enquiry is based on those six monosyllables, and the orderly presentation of a scientific paper is helped by trying to answer the questions.' They can frame the material of not only scientific papers, but also of narrative content, for instance context – the time (when) and place (where) the subject (who) is subjected (what and how). Perhaps Orwell's relativism, his thoughts on the writer's subject matter and motives being framed in the earliest

Table 11.1 Writing a 55-word story

---

1. Identify a compelling story – you have experiences – clinician/patient/ other. Or use prompts (as suggested here).
2. Write down everything.
3. Get the words done – don't edit at this stage, don't pause for the exact word – just write: phrases, words, key chunks of memory.
4. Read what you have written; look for structure – what would you want to convey? Read it out loud.
5. Put away (optional); take a time interval; come back to it – every interval and revision improves the work.
6. Edit. You may need to be ruthless. Restructure. Whole chunks may need to move.
7. Share your work with others for feedback and reactions.
8. Recycle to 4. Edit to 55 words: kernelise.
   A. The title doesn't contribute to word count but should not be more than seven words.
   B. Contractions count as single words.
   C. Eliminating articles can help trim the word count.
9. If the word count is exceeded, you may have material that needs a vehicle other than a 55-word story. As for a 'kill your darling' purple patch that requires (reluctant) excision, it may just belong somewhere else.
10. Formatting is pivotal – experiment with punctuation, sentence anatomy, line length, indentations, white space.

Source: Modified from Fogarty (2010).

of life experiences, is justified (Orwell, 1994). It is interesting that the fundamental cognitive function and basis of mental state examination, orientation, is similarly couched in terms of time (when), place (where), and person (who) (Peer et al., 2015). Further, Beck's cognitive triad for depression invokes negative views of the world: place (where), self (who) and future (time when) (Beck, 1967). Perhaps the very foundation of identity is actually narrative, the stories we tell ourselves.

In Margaret Atwood's 'Five Visits to the Word-Hoard' (Atwood, 2002), what Anglo-Saxon poets called their 'well of inspiration', words being 'seen as a mysterious treasure', she advises us: 'if you're blocked, try changing the tense or the person.' So, again, we are encouraged to manipulate two of the cardinal dials of experience, time and space (place). Furthermore, as observed by Eudora Welty: 'The events in our lives happen in a sequence of time, but in their significance to ourselves, they find their own order ... the continuous thread of revelation' (Welty 1984; Scannell, 2002).

For 55-word stories, Fogarty's second and third injunctions involve starting to write uninhibitedly (Table 11.1). Don't edit, get it written.

Open the word hoard (Bolton, 2005). Sometimes it helps to be primed and prompted.

My English teacher was an eccentric, a brilliant mimic, director of plays and advocate of Dylan Thomas, Yeats and Housman. Alongside his enthusiasm for past masters, he berated us to write short-form fragmentary poetry; he encouraged all to create – to reach within or beyond, and not to worry about any formulaic marking scheme. He believed (as I do not – I am a 'reach within' person) in *inspiration from without*. 'Pen and paper ready, eyes shut' – 27 pairs of eyes shut. He chalked, in his immaculate script, on the board, a message, a 'prompt': 'The Hill' or 'Swan' (or whatever, for there were many). 'Open your eyes – Go'.

In this method, we had a minute for any prompt: look and write. *React!* Give 60 seconds of non-stop writing. *Write!* For now, just react, write fast – faster – keep writing – disjointed – mess – structureless – un-patterned – devolved – skeletal.

Afterwards, you relax and see what you have, and revise, re-order, carve, add, subtract, retract, invert. The method is analogous to Graham's instructions: 'Write a bad version as fast as you can; rewrite it over and over' (Graham, 2005).

My teacher had a kind unassuming editorial hand, encouraging for being in beautifully scripted elegant handwriting. The message (and a lesson should any copyeditor choose to heed it) is that his deliberation said: 'I have taken time to truly read and consider your work'. After the creation, and revisions, and re-revisions, we would read aloud, and debate, and analyse. Then was the time, when we had a clear picture of swans or hills or trees, to get us to read a sentinel piece. These friends are with me still: the arcing aching melancholy and most of the words of Yeats's *The Wild Swans at Coole* (Yeats, 1919).

I reflect on my involvement with the ethically questionable when I read three texts: Williams's 'The Use of Force' (Williams, 1984), Richard Selzer's 'Mercy' (he administers what he deems will be a fatal dose of opiate for escalating severe chronic pain in a patient with pancreatic cancer) and 'Brute' (he sutures the earlobes of a patient to the gurney, to keep him still) (Selzer, 1982). These stories compel an uncomfortable examination of ethical precepts (Hudson-Jones, 1999).

Where does that bring me, in 55 words, following the guide in Table 11.1?

BOX 11.3   MEDICAL STUDENT ELECTIVE: 'GO BROADEN YOUR EXPERIENCE'

Thirty years back, India –
  Dusk and dust
  Drinking chai roadside
  The surgeon nodded:
  The solitary hunched woman in a pink-purple sari
  Hand-tilling this barren field: its indifferent unyielding soil
  '28-years-old, two children – mitral valve is gone – needs replacement'
  'How much?'
  'In Delhi... $400' He shrugged
  'Will charity fund it?'
  'No'
  $400 – same as my airfare

The absence of full stops in this piece is an allusion to Mark Tully's book *No Full Stops in India*, where the opening sentences are: 'How do you cope with the poverty?' That must be the question I have been asked most frequently by visitors to India. I often reply, "I don't have to. The poor do" (Tully, 1991).

Though my teacher used words on the board, perhaps stories and visual art are better prompts; they demand answers from the viewer, serve and return interactions like those we categorise for early childhood, questions–answers–questions …

> *One of the many ways I appreciate the arts is as a source from which questions are generated. To sit quietly with a poem, to stand before an image or installation, to listen to a piece of music, is to open oneself up to both questioning the work and being questioned by it.*

(Okoro, 2022)

In addition to texts, Rita Charon uses paintings and photographs as primers/prompts for thinking about narrative-based medicine and the medical humanities. Her lectures are replete with pictures by Rothko, Cassatt, Van Gogh, Whistler (Charon, 2008), and photographs by Salgado and Sugimoto. In the Whistler picture *Sea and Rain: Variations in Violet and Green* (1865) (Charon, 2008), the translucent figure is knee-deep in the water, confronting the magnitude, and is impermanent before it. In *A Fortunate Man*, the classic book by John Berger and Jean Mohr, the photographs of landscape and people are similarly evocative on an emotional level, and the landscape assumes a historical and personal significance (Berger & Mohr, 1968; Huntley, 2001).

A discussion of possible prompts should also include Brian Eno's Oblique Strategies – which involve directions stimulated at random by drawing a card, when sessions were stalling (Harford, 2016):

> *Be the first not to do what has never not been done before*
> *Emphasise the flaws*
> *Only a part, not the whole*
> *Change instrument roles*
> *Look at the order in which you do things*
> *Twist the spine*

Harford goes on to explain: 'the disruption puts an artist, scientist or engineer in unpromising territory – a deep valley rather than a familiar hilltop. But then expertise kicks in.'

Mood matters too. John Cleese is explicit about the role of mood in influencing thoughts and thereby one's art: 'Your thoughts follow your mood … so obvious. We all know that, if we're depressed, we don't have cheerful, optimistic, energetic thoughts … feeling creative isn't exactly an emotion. It's a frame of mind' (Cleese, 2022).

How does the creative act occur? I am quickly reduced to metaphor, to the picture of the 'Thought Fox' emerging at night and padding its prints across the page (Hughes, 2003). Consider your reaction to a prompt, and the step beyond, the reaction that a reader might have to your piece. Impact is dependent on what the reader brings to the painting, to the novel, to the poem, to the 55-word story. In figurative and abstract art, we may access ourselves; where the orthopaedic surgeon sees a hammer, the psychologist may see rage. We see what we know. At the outset, Rorschach did not see his inkblots as a 'test', but as an experiment, 'a non-judgemental and open-ended investigation into people's ways of seeing' (Searls, 2017). Judkins details the Venus of Milo (Judkins, 2015): though based on an unusual aesthetic dynamic spiral, the statue is 'broken and mutilated', incomplete. The viewer must fill in the gaps. Figurative art is like this: incomplete, perhaps flawed or broken, perhaps in progress. As with diamonds, the flaws give the colour.

BOX 11.4

Instruction: Get five sheets of paper, and a pen and ink or pencil.

Developing the idea of pictures as prompts, here are figurative works by Lucas Seymour.

All you need to respond is volition, pencil or ink, and paper. The next pages are a picture apiece. Turn the page, look and write.

Fifty-five words are all I ask of you. You may find, limited to 55 words, a tendency to abstraction and rhythm that renders your piece poetic. Writing (as if) for publication is the right aim. It encourages reaction, discussion, revision, improvement and learning, thereby. But I know the value of the unpublished fragmentary typescripts on the corkboard above my desk; the short statement of resilience, the motif-experience, the melancholy given shape. For writers, 'it helps to have a broad base of knowledge that extends beyond the boundaries of literature' (Csikszentmihalyi, 1996). Here again, we in healthcare are ideally placed. We are given a passport to so many bodies and so many stories.

When you try, I don't know if you will reach within (introspection) or without (the great beyond). Prompts, textual or visual, might stimulate either. But looking 'without' presupposes a 'within'. And possibly the reverse. So, we may uncover, or discover ... Storr has this to say on narrative and psychological depth:

> The lesson of story is that we have no idea how wrong we are. Discovering the fragile parts of our neural models means listening for their cry. When we become irrationally emotional and defensive, we're often betraying the parts of us that require the most aggressive protection.
>
> (Storr, 2019)

Before you turn the page: anticipate the reveal of the warped tarot. Go! Turn the card, turn the page.

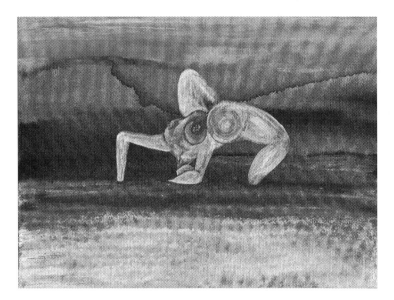

Figure 11.2

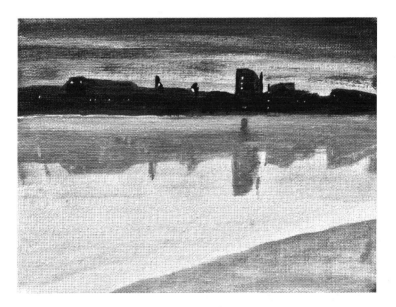

Figure 11.3

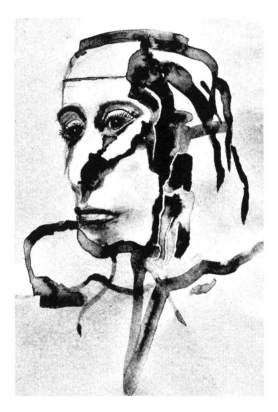

Figure 11.4

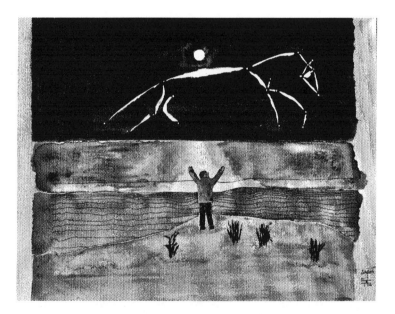

Figure 11.5

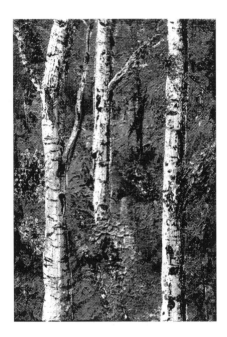

Figure 11.6

This quasi-instructional chapter has had meandering paths; I wander in the woods. I am in a clearing now. Above all, you should write. Here are two eloquent advocates for writing and art:

> *Life is sometimes hard. Things go wrong, in life and in love and in business and in friendship and in health and in all the other ways that life can go wrong. And when things get tough, this is what you should do ... MAKE GOOD ART. I'm serious.*

> (Gaiman, 2018)

In *The War of Art*: 'Creative work is not a selfish act or a bid for attention ... Don't cheat us of your contribution. Give us what you've got (Pressfield, 2012).

★★★

I ask: 'What were the major things that upset you in what I said?'

He shakes his head.

I am okay with silence, but after an appropriate few seconds – of consideration – I say gently: 'That's a lot of information to take on in one go. We can talk about this another time.'

I pause again: 'I wonder, would it make sense for you to write things down ... what worries you, what you can't say? What has upset you?'

Now he looks up at me, eyes to eyes, as if to defend his writing from my prying.

'Dr Jim. I write, not to immerse myself in the here and now, but to *escape* my reality.'

REFERENCES AND FURTHER READING

Adair J. Reading to generate ideas. Chapter 10. In: *The art of creative thinking*. Kogan Page Ltd; 2007, pp. 51–5.

Antoniou S.A., Antoniou G.A., Granderath F.A., Mavroforou A., Giannoukas A.D., Antoniou A.I. Reflections of the Hippocratic oath in modern medicine. *World J. Surg.* 2010; *34*: 3075–9.

Asher R. Aren't I lucky? I can write! In: *Talking sense about medicine*. London: Psychology News Press; 2015a, pp. 219–26.

Asher R. Six honest serving men for medical writers. In: *Talking sense about medicine*. London: Psychology News Press; 2015b, pp. 60–76.

Atwood M. Five visits to the word-hoard. In: *Burning Questions*. London: Chatto & Windus; 2002, pp. 37–48.

Atwood M. Introduction: Into the labyrinth. In: *On writers and writing*. Virago Press; 2003a, pp. xiii–xxii.

Atwood M. Descent: Negotiating with the dead. Chapter 6. In: *On writers and writing*. Virago Press; 2003b, pp. 137–61.

Beck A.T. *The diagnosis and management of depression*. Philadelphia, PA: University of Pennysylvania Press; 1967.

Beaulieu M.D. Make a difference: Become a positive deviant. *Can. Fam. Physician* 2013; *59*: 447.

Berger J. *Ways of seeing*. London: BBC and Penguin; 1972.

Berger J., Mohr J. *A fortunate man*. Readers Union edition. London: Penguin Press; 1968.

Berkowitz I., McCarthy C., eds. *Innovation with information technologies in healthcare*. London: Springer; 2013.

Bolton G. Opening the word hoard. *J Med. Ethics: Medical Humanities* 2005; *31*: 43–9.

Caban-Martinez A.J., Garcia Beltran W.F. Advancing medicine one research note at a time: The educational value in clinical case reports. *BMC Res. Notes* 2012; *5*: 293.

Charon R. The art of medicine: Narrative evidence based medicine. *Lancet*. 2008; *371*: 296–7.

Childress M.D. In the literature. *AMA J. Ethics* 2017; *19*: 272–80.

Christianson A.L. More stories. *JAMA* 2002; *288*: 931.

Cleese J. *Creativity*. Penguin Books; 2022.

Csikszentmihalyi M. The domain of the word. Chapter 10. In: *Creativity*. New York: HarperCollins; 1996, pp. 237–64.

Dominiczak M.H. Sir William Osler. *Clin. Chem.* 2014; *60*: 800–1.

Elwood M. One hundred and ten basic ideas for short shorts. Chapter 20. In: *Write the short short*. The Writer Inc Publishers; 1947, pp. 210–41.

Fogarty C.T. Fifty-five word stories: 'Small jewels' for personal reflection and teaching. *Fam. Med.* 2010; *42*: 400–2.

Fogarty C.T. Why I write. *Fam. Med.* 2013; *45*: 52–3.

Fogarty C.T., Bogar C.B., Costello P., Greenfield G.W., Neely K. 55-word stories: A collection from the 32nd forum for behavioural science in family medicine. *Fam. Med.* 2013; *45*: 656–7.

Gaiman N. Make good art. Chapter 3. In: *Art Matters*. Headline Publishing Group; 2018, pp. 47–97.

Gardner M. *Undiluted hocus-pocus*. Oxford: Princeton University Press, 2013.

Gawande A. *Better: A surgeon's notes on performance*. New York: Picador; 2007.

Gawande A. The bell curve. *New Yorker* 2004; *6*: 82–9.

Geyman J.P. Why do we write? *Fam. Med.* 2013; *45*: 40–1.

Graham P. *Writing, briefly*. paulgraham.com 2005 (accessed 7 November 2022).

Graham P. *Putting ideas into words*. paulgraham.com 2022 (accessed 7 November 2022).

Grant W.D. Life in 55 words: part 1. *Fam. Med.* 2008; *40*: 241–4.

Green B. Use of the Hippocratic or other professional oaths in UK medical schools in 2017: Practice, perception of benefit and principlism. *BMC Res. Notes* 2017; *10*: 777.

Harford T. Creativity. Chapter 1. In: *Messy*. Abacus; 2016, pp. 7–35.

Hein P. *Collected Grooks I*. Copenhagen, Denmark: Piet Hein Publishing; 2002.

Hicks J. A poet with a slide rule: Piet Hein bestrides art and science. *Life Magazine*, 14 October 1966: 55–66.

Holub M. The rules of writing short columns. In: *The Jingle Bell principle*. Newcastle: Bloodaxe Books Ltd; 1992, pp. 7–8.

Hudson-Jones A. Narrative in medical ethics. *BMJ* 1999; *318*: 253–6.

Hughes T. The thought fox. In: *Collected poems*. London: Faber & Faber Ltd; 2003.

Hulkower R. The history of the Hippocratic oath: Outdated, inauthentic, and yet still relevant. *Einstein J. Biol. Med.* 2016; *25*: 41–4.

Huntley J.S. In search of a fortunate man. *Lancet* 2001; *357*: 546–9.

Huntley J.S. Castell Coch. *J. Roy. Soc. Med.* 2004; *97*: 90–2.

Judkins R. If it ain't broke, break it. In: *The art of creative thinking*. London: Sceptre, Hodder & Stoughton Ltd: 2015, pp. 65–8.

Kipling R. The elephant's child. In: *Just so stories*. London: Macmillan & Co; 1902.

Laverty R., Anvari A., Polmear M., Qureshi U. 55-word stories about medical student's clerkship experiences. *Mil. Med.* 2017; *182*: 1744.

McPhee J. *Draft No. 4: On the writing process*. New York: Farrar, Straus & Giroux; 2017.

Moran J. *First you write a sentence: The elements of reading, writing… and life*. Penguin Random House; 2018.

Moss S. *The world's shortest stories*. Philadelphia, PA: Running Press; 1995.

Okoro E. The power of a good question. Life and arts, 6 August 2022, *Weekend Financial Times*.

Orwell G. Why I write. Essay 1. In: G. Orwell. Essays. London: Penguin Books; 1994, pp. 1–6.

Osler W. *The quotable Osler*. Philadelphia, PA: American College of Physicians; 2003.

Peer M., Salomon R., Goldberg I., Blanke O., Arzy S. Brain system for mental orientation in space, time, and person. *Proc. Natl. Acad. Sci. USA* 2015; *112*: 11072–7.

Peterkin A. Practical strategies for practising narrative-based medicine. *Can. Fam. Physician* 2012; *58*: 63–4.

Pressfield S. *The war of art*. New York: Black Irish Entertainment LLC; 2012.

Python M. *Monty Python's big red book*. London: Methuen; 1971.

Scannell K. Writing for our lives: Physician narratives and medical practice. *Ann. Int. Med.* 2002; *137*: 779–81.

Scheetz A., Fry M.E. The stories. *JAMA* 2000; *283*: 1934.

Searls D. *The inkblots*. London: Simon & Schuster; 2017.

Selzer R. Brute. *New Engl. Rev.* (1978–82) 1981; *4*: 2–5.

Selzer R. *Letters to a young doctor*. New York: Touchstone Books; 1982.

Stein H.F. Why I write: Reflections from 40 years of clinical teaching and writing. *Fam. Med.* 2013; *45*: 46–7.

Storr W. Plots, endings and meanings. Chapter 4. In: *The science of storytellling*. London: William Collins; 2019, pp. 177–203.

Tully M. *No full stops in India*. London: Penguin Books; 1991.

Welty E. One writer's beginnings. In: *The William E. Massey St. Lectures in the history of American civilisation, 1983*. PR: Harvard University Press; 1984, pp. 68–9.

Williams W.C. *The doctor stories*. New York: New Directions; 1984.

Yeats W.B. *The wild swans at Coole*. London: Macmillan; 1919.

FIGURE LEGENDS

Figure 11.2 Eve (2022. Lucas Seymour. Acrylic on canvas)

Figure 11.3 Estuary (2022. Lucas Seymour. Acrylic on canvas)

Figure 11.4 Stare (2021. Lucas Seymour. Mixed media on paper)

Figure 11.5 Starhorse (2022. Lucas Seymour. Acrylic on canvas)

Figure 11.6 Aspen (2022. Lucas Seymour. Acrylic on canvas)

THE END OF THE STORY?

Colin Robertson and Fiona Nicol

Unless we can devise ways to get people to talk about how they want to live while they are dying, our efforts … will be like groping in the dark.

Leadbeater and Garber, *Dying for Change*, 2010

THE FIVE STORIES OF DEATH

For many the thought that, one day, we will no longer exist is terrifying. Accordingly, death denial is common – a conscious refusal to approach and openly discuss the process and mechanisms involved. For some, denial reflects that death itself is unimaginable.

It appears to me impossible that I should cease to exist, or that this active, restless spirit, equally alive to joy and sorrow, should only be organised dust – ready to fly abroad the moment the spring snaps, or the spark goes out, which kept it together.

(Mary Wollstonecraft)

The philosopher Stephen Cave thinks that one way of managing the fear of death is to tell stories about it. He suggests that humans have told themselves these stories throughout different times and cultures to comfort ourselves and that these can be categorised in one of five ways.

DOI: 10.1201/9781003409151-12

BOX 12.1 THE FIVE STORIES OF DEATH

- The Elixir story
- The Resurrection story
- The Soul story
- The Legacy story
- The Wisdom story

The first, he calls the Elixir story: in this, a magic pill, potion, spell or rite wards off illness or ageing and avoids death. Few people believe in magic, but these ideas are still prevalent, and age also appears to affect these attitudes (Maxfield et al., 2007): 'I am young, don't smoke, eat oat bran, take exercise and my statin – I don't have to think about death.'

Of course, our real experience of elixirs of life, in whatever form they are taken, fails to match their promise. This means that we need a backup plan. Cave calls this the Resurrection story: this promises that your physical or conscious self can be restored to life after death. For some, a promised afterlife is the principal focus of their religion. Their actions in life are dedicated and directed to its attainment. Jesus's story was not the first god figure to be resurrected. The Egyptian gods were mummified to help them to the afterlife and now we have novel technologies to support and even replace belief. Cryonics is the low-temperature preservation of humans who cannot be sustained by contemporary medicine, with the hope that in the future, technology will enable healing and resuscitation to be possible.

Most people believe that they have a soul or spirit – a form of immortal essence – and that even if the previous stories do not work out, they may live on because this is reborn in some form. The Soul story is Cave's third story; the early Christians believed in a physical afterlife but as time went on and the final judgement did not happen, they started to change the story into one where the afterlife was metaphysical. Other religions share similar ideas: Buddhists believe in the concept of an essence being reincarnated even if not necessarily in human form. For Hindus, an individual's spirit is permanent, and reincarnation allows repeated rebirth. The era of the computer has further contributed to these views. Even if physical restoration is not contemplated, 'consciousness' may be: 'My brain will be uploaded into the internet or onto a "chip".'

The fourth story is Legacy: the ideas live on through the work you have done or through your children and therefore your genes. Certainly, we return to atoms and molecules, and these will 'live on' as matter/energy can neither be created nor destroyed.

It won't be nothing. We'll be alive again in a thousand blades of grass, and a million leaves; we'll be falling in the raindrops and blowing in the fresh breeze; we'll be glittering in the dew under the stars and the moon out there in the physical world.

(Philip Pullman)

For some, this form of 'afterlife', even though it contains nothing of their physical or spiritual nature, is reassuring.

Considerable evidence suggests that previous generations and other cultures believed in one of these stories. The Pyramids of Egypt and the Neolithic tombs such as Göbekli Tepe in Turkey, Maes Howe in Orkney and Newgrange in Ireland are atmospheric and enigmatic. The Romans had the Parentalia, a nine-day festival where families visited the tombs of relations, offering meals to the dead and having a celebratory picnic often in a specially constructed room within the tomb itself. Each year, three million visitors stand in front of the Taj Mahal, possibly forgetting that it was built as a mausoleum for Mumtaz Mahal by her husband Shah Jahan. The Victorian pre-occupation with death and mourning still resonates in architecture, monuments, art and flaking gravestones in increasingly overgrown graveyards. Visit the Glasgow Necropolis or Kensal Green cemetery in London to see extraordinary examples of nineteenth-century Cities of the Dead.

Cave's point is that these recurring stories arise from our fear of death and non-existence. He suggests a fifth approach, the Wisdom story, in which, since we do not know what death is like, there is nothing to fear. Essentially, it means do not waste time worrying about your time being limited but accept every moment as if it were an unexpected gift or an incredible stroke of luck – which, of course, it is. Think where and when you could have been born and marvel that you have the opportunities that you have had and will continue to have. Earlier philosophers have had similar views:

While we are, death is not; when death is come, we are not. Death is thus of no concern either to the living or to the dead.

(Epicurus)

And if this seems too challenging to contemplate, then consider Montaigne:

We do not know where death awaits us: so let us wait for it everywhere … Life has no evil for him who had thoroughly understood that loss of life is not an evil.

THE ACT OF DYING

All these stories refer to death itself and not the act of dying, yet, historically, discussing death openly included pragmatic advice on how to die. *Seppuku* – a ritual suicide originally retained for Japanese samurai – was an extreme form. In medieval Europe the Black Death stimulated the publication of guides to death. The *Tractus artis bene moriendi* (A treatise on the art of a good death) was commissioned by the Council of Constance in 1414–1418. The abbreviated, illustrated version, *Ars Moriendi*, provided a practical template for (Christian) death, including: why death is inevitable; questions to ask the dying; advice on managing the death etc. (Figure 12.1). These books were extremely popular, were translated into many European languages and initiated a series of similar texts culminating in 1651 with Jeremy Taylor's poetic 'The Rules and Exercises of Holy Dying'.

In contrast, our twenty-first-century experience of death is muted and remote, despite our daily media exposure to graphic images of violence and death, real and fictional. Very few modern-day Westerners have actually seen, let alone touched, a dead body. This contrasts sharply with the numbers of deaths seen on television, films and video games by children up to the age of 18 which number the tens of thousands. More than 95% of these deaths involve violence and involve young or middle-aged adults. But reality is very different. Approximately half a million people die each year in the UK. Of these, two-thirds are over 75 years and one-third are over 85 years. Three-quarters of these deaths are 'predictable' in that they follow a period of chronic illness or decline (Leadbeater & Garber, 2010). Fewer than 1% of us will die by being shot, stabbed, blown up, bisected by laser beams or exsanguinated by vampires in the manner seen on screen. So, for most of the population, the true causes of death – cancer, cardio- and cerebro-vascular disease and dementia – are unrecognised. More importantly, the mechanism of death is poorly appreciated and certainly has little in common with its onscreen portrayal.

LIFE-SAVING OR DEATH-DELAYING?

There are essentially four modes of dying (Figure 12.2): sudden (usually unexpected) death, for example due to a cardiac arrest, major intracranial haemorrhage, accident or suicide; terminal illness, such as cancer or infection; organ failure where one system after another stops working; and frailty, with a slow decline where the individual progressively loses the ability to function and look after themselves. The first two modes proportionately affect younger, more than older, people. Organ failure can affect any age, but the reality is that most of us will die through frailty and old age.

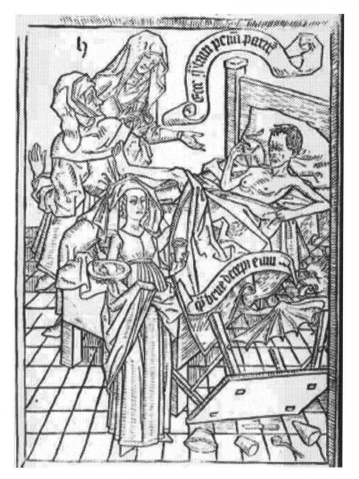

Figure 12.1 Woodcut from *Ars Moriendi*. (From: http://userpage.fu-berlin.de/
~aeimhof/seelefr.htm.)

Nowadays, we talk a lot about life-saving interventions and drugs
but surely we mean death-delaying? Nothing will ever actually stop
people from eventually dying. So if we cannot control the fact that
we will die then can we control the mode of our dying? Medicine
has made major contributions to this situation. Trying to prolong
an active, sentient and fulfilled life is admirable, but there must be a
limit. Fortunately, we cannot delay or suspend death forever. True
immortality would be insufferable. In the Greek myths, the Trojan
Tithonos and more recently Captain Jack Harkness, from the *Doctor
Who* spin-off *Torchwood*, experience all of the pain and distress that
true immortality would entail.

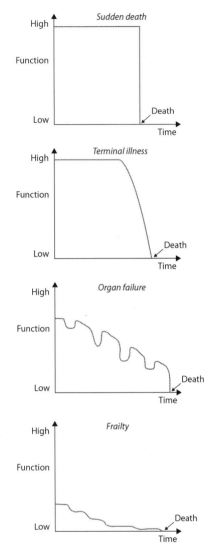

Figure 12.2 The modes of death.

Perhaps the best approach is to consider death in narrative terms as one end to a story – by its presence, enabling a true appreciation of life.

THE PORNOGRAPHY OF DEATH

Death replaced the Victorian taboo subjects of sex and birth in twentieth-century Western society (Gorer, 1955). By 'pornography',

Table 12.1 Euphemisms for death

- Angels carried them away
- Asleep
- Bought (it, a one-way ticket, the farm)
- Breathed their last
- Brown bread (probably cockney rhyming slang – bread = dead)
- Cashed or checked in (or out)
- Ceased to be
- Checked into the horizontal Hilton
- Climbed the stairway to heaven
- Croaked
- *Deceased*
- Departed
- Entered (the Pearly Gates, eternal rest, the hereafter, Heaven etc.)
- Faded away
- Fallen off their perch (cf. Monty Python and the 'Dead Parrot sketch')
- Flatlined
- Gave up the ghost
- Got their just reward (or wings)
- *Gone* or *Went* (West, to a better place, toes up, to join the ancestors, the way of all flesh, to their maker, to be with the Lord, to Davy Jones's locker, to the happy Hunting grounds, to their Long Home etc.)
- Hopped the twig
- Journey's end
- Kicked (the bucket, can)
- Knocked on Heaven's door
- Laid down
- Left or Lost (this life)
- Left the building (Elvis has …)
- Met (an untimely end, their Maker)
- *Passed* (away, on, the point of no return)
- Pegged out
- Perished
- Playing a harp
- Popped their clogs
- Pushing up daisies
- Resting (in peace)
- Shuffled off this mortal coil (*Hamlet* Act III, scene i)
- Six feet under (the traditional depth for burial)
- Sleeps (with the fishes)
- *Slipped* (away, their cable)
- Substantive negative outcome
- Succumbed
- Surrendered their life
- Terminated
- Turned up their toes
- Their number's up
- Walked the plank
- Was called home

Note: The more common UK terms are in italics.

Gorer meant that talking about death produces shock, disquiet or social embarrassment. Today, most people find it far easier to talk about sex than death and have had greater first-hand exposure to it. Our reluctance to discuss death has elements of magical thinking. This is when a person attributes an effect in reality to a thought or unconnected event (Bolton et al., 2002). Magical thinking is a normal developmental stage in young children, but many adults have similar convictions (Wooley, 1997; Evans, 2002). There is no difference between the pre-school child who refuses to stand on the cracks between paving stones and the tennis or football star who must repeat a fixed ritual before serving or taking a penalty kick. Adults who reject talking about death may believe that death may be precipitated simply by mentioning it.

There are a multitude of euphemisms for death (Table 12.1). This is the true 'pornography' of death. Euphemisms sanitise and obscure reality. If we use these terms, we collude in the deception and may cause misunderstanding. Telling a relative that someone in the intensive care unit has 'gone to a better place', may be misconstrued as them having been returned to the general surgical ward.

The combative language often used to describe dying is also striking. Popular obituaries and eulogies regularly use emotive words like 'battle', 'fight', 'struggle' and 'combat' in relation to the terminal disease. This military language is very strange. Is it accurate or appropriate? Since death is inevitable, while individual 'battles' may be won they can only be skirmishes in a campaign doomed to fail. Do so many people really 'fight' terminal conditions or is this simply a reflection of their clinicians and carers rejecting a natural process. Maybe the 'fight' is against the dying process rather than death as a state.

Age appears to affect attitudes to death (Maxfield et al., 2007). Young adults rationalise and implicitly reject the possibility: 'I am young, fit, don't smoke, eat healthily, take exercise so I don't have to think about death for many years to come.' Increasing age, with greater experience of death, is often accompanied by acceptance of death.

STORY BOX 12.2

Miss Fisken was 92 and had been a very sprightly patient of mine for many years. She lived in private sheltered housing by herself, had never had any serious illness or been admitted to hospital. I hardly ever saw her in the health centre. The request for a house call suggested a serious problem. When I arrived, she was lying in bed with her face to the wall. Her friend told me that she had not heard from Miss Fisken for some time and had called round to find her in bed and with no food in the house. She appeared quite alert, had been managing to toilet herself and was very concerned at her friend asking me to attend.

I could find no acute symptoms or change in her mental state, but she told me that she was now ready to die. She refused to consider that her decision was irrational, was not depressed and had no symptoms of mental illness. Indeed, her decision that now was the time for her to die seemed, on the face of it, to be quite rational and well considered. She told me that all her friends, except the lady who had let me in, were dead. She had no family and no one to leave her possessions to. We discussed what she might do with them as she had many historical artefacts that may have been of interest to certain museums. No one could accuse her of not being of sound mind. She had become increasingly frail and had not been out for some time before her friend called.

So she turned her face to the wall, metaphorically as well as literally and after about ten days died peacefully in her own bed. The district nurses had attended to her, and I visited daily to see whether she required something for any symptoms, but she never did. She did not seem to suffer pain or thirst. She drank what she felt she needed. One morning shortly before she died, she seemed to be sleeping and I gently touched her shoulder. She opened her eyes and seeing me, groaned and asked:

'Am I still here, doctor? I had no idea it would take so long.'

'To be honest – neither did I,' I replied.

Older adults seem to have more balanced, positive and less aggressive coping methods (Diehl et al., 1996; Heckstein & Schulz, 1995). This may be the consequence of higher levels of positive affect and lower levels of negative affect seen in older adults, reflected in their greater contentment, and less anxiety and depression (Mroczek & Kolarz, 1998; Lawton et al., 1993). However, age and physical health may bear little relation to the acceptance of death. The Epicurean epitaph: *Non fui, fui, non sum, non curo* (I was not; I was; I am not; I care not), carved on many Roman memorials is sometimes used today at humanist funerals but there are many who will not 'Go gentle into that good night' but will 'rage, rage against the dying of the light' (Dylan Thomas).

STORY BOX 12.3 A PANDEMIC STORY

I am 72 years old. I am dying. I am very angry. I write this to help my anger.

I knew my diagnosis. I had been a surgeon for 40 years. I phoned and tried to get an appointment with my family doctor. I couldn't get beyond the receptionist. Eventually, after three calls, I spoke with him and said what was wrong. Without seeing me in person 'because of the infection risk', blood tests and an ultrasound scan were arranged. I indicated that neither was likely to be of help and that if a diagnosis was to be confirmed then a CT scan was more appropriate. No luck. After two inconclusive ultrasounds and another six weeks, a CT was performed and confirmed my diagnosis. I was referred to a surgical consultant whom I had trained 20 years earlier. This was my first actual contact with a clinician. She examined me carefully and showed me the scan. We agreed that surgery was not indicated, and my life expectancy was likely to be weeks.

I live alone and went home. I wept for the first time in 65 years. My niece visits daily, which is against the guidance, but who cares. My family doctor has still not visited, but arranged for a palliative care nurse to come. She is wonderful. She takes off her mask and talks with me.

Why am I so angry? In part, at the failings of my body – I am now incontinent, which is unbelievably distressing. But mainly my anger is at my former profession. The pandemic has been an excuse for some to distance themselves from their patients. Some of my elderly friends have had much worse experiences than mine – I grieve for them.

Healthcare workers do not necessarily have a greater understanding of death than patients and their relatives and are often ill-equipped to advise, direct or educate them. Too often, we focus on restoring and maintaining health. For many doctors, even the physical experience of death is remote. Medical students used to spend their first two years in regular contact with a formalin-soaked body in the dissecting room and recently deceased bodies in the post-mortem suite. Both experiences are now rare. Dissection has become prosection. Autopsy has been replaced by digital imaging and 3-D colour reconstruction. There is no connection between seeing or handling a dissected limb or a dead body and looking at a computer-generated image. Death has become a video game.

Although undergraduates are taught how to break bad news compassionately, we don't impart an appreciation of the limits of medical care and confront the inevitability of death. It is very difficult to avoid colluding in death denial unless we have a mentor who shows us how to recognise the limits of modern medicine's competence and support patients in this.

THE QUALITY OF DEATH

In the UK, the majority of deaths occur in hospital – increasingly in an intensive care or high dependency unit, with the patient surrounded, distanced and isolated by sophisticated expensive equipment. This is despite the fact that nearly 60% of the population is scared of dying in hospital, let alone the monetary cost to an increasingly cash-strapped NHS. The technology provides a carapace for the staff but excludes or even threatens relatives. Why do so many people die in hospital since two-thirds of us want to die at home? Death produces fear; we are most scared of 'being told we are dying' (71% very or fairly scared), 'dying alone' (65%), 'having a close friend or family member dying' (79%) and of dying 'in pain' (80%) (First national VOICES survey of bereaved people, 2012, Dying Matters Survey, 2014).

Most people would choose to 'die in their sleep' or have a sudden death, most often from unheralded cardiac arrest, cerebrovascular event or trauma, as their preferred mode of death. While this avoids pain or suffering, it may only be best for everyone if they have already said all they would wish to their family and friends, organised all their financial affairs, planned their funeral arrangements and are fully prepared for death itself. But few of us live each day as if it were the last. Despite the ready availability of templates and good practical advice from organisations such as the Patient's Association and Age UK, a minority have made advance directives or living wills (www .patients-association.org.uk; www.ageuk.org.uk).

Richard Smith, a former editor of the *British Medical Journal*, wrote a blog for the journal titled 'Dying of cancer is the best death'. Unsurprisingly, with this label, there were many angry and distressed responses from readers – most from members of the public. The most vociferous reactions were from patients with cancer, or relatives or friends of individuals who had died of cancer. It is instructive to read these comments. Many include one or more of the reactions first highlighted by Elisabeth Kübler-Ross: denial, anger, bargaining, depression, acceptance (Kübler-Ross, 2014). A common underlying thread was that the writers had experienced some, or all, of the components of a 'bad' death. Intolerable or uncontrolled pain and cancer deaths in children or young people were particularly highlighted. But Smith's central point was misunderstood. The real message was that often a diagnosis of cancer provides the patient and their family a measure of time. Irrespective of its duration, this can allow a degree of preparation and the achievement of some, hopefully all, of the components of a 'good death' (Table 12.2). By contrast, sudden, unexpected death robs the patient, and especially their family, of this.

Table 12.2 Possible components of 'bad' and 'good' deaths

Possible components of a 'bad' death	Possible components of a 'good' death
Uncontrolled or severe pain	Having those you wish (family, friends) around
Uncontrolled symptoms e.g. nausea, dyspnoea, constipation	Pain-free
	Having dignity
	Not protracted
Being lonely	Having control
Stigmatised condition e.g. HIV	Being perceived as a unique and whole individual
	Prepared for death (where I wish to die, funeral arrangements, what to expect regarding care etc.)
Loss of dignity or privacy	Dying at the 'right' time
Unprepared, unresolved issues	Completion (issues of faith, resolution of conflicts)
	Ability to contribute to others e.g. gifts, information, time

Source: Adapted from: Smith, 2000; A Good Death: NHS Public Health North East, 2010; Costello, 2006; Steinhauser et al., 2000.

STORY BOX 12.4

Mr Urquhart had lived and worked for many years in Africa. He had developed a rectal cancer and had surgery while still there. He and his wife returned to the UK and bought a flat at the top of four flights of steep stone stairs in an old part of the city. There was no lift. They both came to openly discuss their plans as he had hoped to have several years before the cancer caught up with him; it was not to be.

He had intense pain from bony secondaries and local invasion of the pelvis, and immobility very quickly became a problem. He and his wife wanted him to die at home. They bore their altered circumstances with remarkable stoicism and an unusual openness. He never complained but would simply say that the painkillers were 'not quite up to the mark'. In spite of the involvement of the local hospice and their expertise, the only thing that worked to keep his pain under any sort of control was subcutaneous morphine. I was pregnant at the time and arrived daily at the top of the stairs carrying my doctor's bag very out of breath. In spite of his situation, they were solicitous about my welfare. Was this a way of deflecting attention from their situation? Perhaps, but they also never avoided discussing what was happening and preparing for it.

Despite our best attempts, pain control was never totally successful; I learned never to promise to control all symptoms. Many people are not just afraid of death but of the process of dying itself, and for some that may be their main fear. His wife remained my patient and often brought me back mementoes of her latest foreign trip. I had become part of their family's story.

Controlling symptoms is only one part of attending the dying. Part of achieving a 'good' death involves temporal prognostication. At the time of diagnosis, patients and their relatives commonly ask for accurate prediction of the time remaining before death. Every clinician has experienced the embarrassment that inaccuracy brings to this discussion: overestimation of the time to death may leave the patient and their family feeling deceived or cheated of time. Underestimation provokes questions as to the accuracy of the diagnosis and the competency of the clinician. Either way, some of the reciprocal trust in the relationship is lost. In one-third of cancer cases, even 'experts' make significant errors of clinical prediction – a 'significant' error being defined as more than half, or double, the eventual survival time. For other terminal conditions, such as heart failure, chronic pulmonary or liver disease, accurate prognostication is even more difficult.

A variety of prognostic tools commonly involving multivariant analysis such as the Palliative Prognostic score (PaP), Palliative Prognostic Index (PPI), Survival Prediction Score (SPS) etc. may be used, but are imperfect. Applied to a 'population', they are helpful, but much less so when discussing the situation with an individual patient, especially as with older patients concomitant illness (e.g. metastatic cancer and chronic pulmonary disease) are likely to be present (Chow et al., 2001; Brandt et al., 2006; Maltoni et al., 2005; Pocock et al., 2013). The situation is exacerbated when decisions are needed regarding the need for, and timing of, palliative or hospice care.

STORY BOX 12.5

James was like a character from Grassic Gibbon's Scottish classic, *Sunset Song*. He was a farmer's son and had no surviving family. He lived for his dog. He presented with seizures and headache. The scan showed a space-occupying lesion, highly suggestive of glioblastoma, in the dominant frontal lobe.

After debulking surgery and radiotherapy, he had a good remission. The histology was typical and confirmed a malignant glioblastoma. At the monthly case review, surgeons, pathologists, radiotherapists and oncologists all agreed on an average survival of about 18 months. In due course he relapsed and had further surgery. Steroids and morphine helped the headaches, but after discussion with James it was agreed to 'wind down' the drugs. He wanted to die 'at home with his dog'. I phoned James's GP for advice about nursing or palliative care in his area. The GP served a small rural community and said that there was little available. 'How long will he survive?' he asked. I thought a few weeks at most. The GP said: 'We have a spare room. If it's only for a few weeks, we could take him and his dog.' The GP's wife was a former nurse and agreed to the plan. 'What saints!' I thought.

Ten years later, Jimmy and his dog were still a part of his doctor's family. The scans and histology were checked repeatedly and independently; slides sent to other centres gave the same diagnosis and prognosis.

James died after 15 years in his doctor's household. His grave is on a quiet clifftop. The stone and its carved inscription were commissioned by his doctor's family.

All of these discussions are compounded if the clinician is uncomfortable with handing over the care and responsibility for a patient in whom they feel they have 'failed'. Irrespective of how and when this conversation takes place the facts must be accurate. The time trajectory of the illness is very helpful, but having these discussions with incomplete information will inevitably lead to problems (see Story Box 12.6).

STORY BOX 12.6

The registrar asked the patient if I could examine the lump in her groin and motioned me forward. The patient, an elderly, uncomplaining, cheery nun from an enclosed order, consented: 'We all have to learn.' The lump was about 2 cm diameter, hard, craggy and fixed; even to an inexperienced medical student its nature was clear.

'I think, if you agree, that we should remove the lump and see what it is,' said the registrar. A biopsy date was set.

'Why didn't you tell her what it must be?' I asked over coffee, full of undergraduate concepts of openness and honesty with patients. 'How would it help her at this stage,' he replied, 'Let's get the pathology first.'

I went to theatre two days later to see the procedure. The registrar expertly dissected the lump out from a mass of fibrous tissue, laid it in a kidney dish and closed the wound. Before putting the specimen into the pathology container, he carefully incised the lump. The scalpel grated on the mass and halted. Gently, he dissected back the fibrous tissue, revealing a dull shiny metal fragment.

On the evening post-operative ward round we stopped at the elderly nun's bed. She was sitting up, drinking tea, taking a lively interest in her companion patients.

'Have you ever had an operation before?' the registrar asked.

'Not really,' she replied.

'What do you mean, "Not really"?'

'Well, in 1940, I went for an operation on my varicose veins. But it was during the Blitz, and they had to stop the operation because the hospital and the operating theatre were bombed. Afterwards, I thought a varicose vein was too trivial to bother about when so many people were badly injured and in need of hospital.'

The registrar looked at me meaningfully and grinned at the nun.

'Well, you don't have to worry about the lump at all. In the chaos of the bombing, they must have left the end of a little instrument called a vein stripper in there. Over time some fibrous tissue grew around it, making it more obvious. Now it's all gone.'

'Oh,' she exclaimed with a twinkle, 'I suppose you could say it's a case of "The Nun and the Stripper".'

NARRATIVE AND A 'GOOD' DEATH

Discussions with a patient about the diagnosis and prognosis of a terminal illness, or informing relatives of a sudden death, are perhaps the greatest communication challenges experienced by clinicians. Some of the obstacles have been mentioned: diagnostic or prognostic uncertainty; feelings of clinician failure; lack of communication training (Finlay & Casarett, 2009).

The clinician may have insufficient experience or incomplete strategies to handle the emotional impact on the patient, relatives or, indeed, themselves. A handy box of tissues is useful, but not enough. The time commitment required may be considerable; matching the pace of the narrative to the participant's needs is critical. Several time periods over days or weeks are likely to be needed. Finally, your cultural, personal or religious beliefs must not intrude upon those of your patient or relatives. This is where the techniques of the actor and performer discussed in Chapter 6 are central. An actor may play parts or say lines with which they deeply disagree, but their audience must implicitly believe in them. Similarly, a musician's façade must prevent, at least during the time of playing, their own emotion inhibiting the performance.

A useful framework for the conduct of these discussions is the SPIKES protocol:

Setting	Ensure privacy, no interruptions, sufficient time.
	Who should be present?
	Have you got all the information necessary e.g. laboratory/scan data etc.?
Perception	What does the patient understand about their disease and current situation?
Information	In what form, and to what extent does the patient wish to receive the information?
Knowledge	Give information clearly, slowly, without jargon and appropriate to the patient's ability and preferences.
	Check repeatedly that they understand what you are saying.
Empathy	Acknowledge the patient's feelings.
Summarise	Review and recheck their understanding.
	What are their goals?
	Establish a plan for follow-up and regular contact.

Source: Adapted from Finlay & Casarett, 2009.

An often-overlooked component is that the patient will have their own stories to tell. A terminal diagnosis, or discussion of death, 'tears the coherence of the life narrative, disrupting daily activities, identities and imagined futures' (Romanoff & Thomson, 2006). For some, particularly the elderly, the need will be to look back and re-evaluate. Here our task is simply to enable the storyteller to tell their stories. The factual accuracy and the coherence of the narrative are less important than the ability to construct and share their tales. How can the accuracy of the information given, by all the participants, be improved? One way is to record the discussion so that the messages can be replayed later to improve understanding. Smartphones and mini-recorders make this simple. Although controversial, a review of recording consultations (although not necessarily in the context of terminal illness) showed that patients valued these recordings, which improved their comprehension and enabled their family to share the information (Elwyn and Buckman, 2015; Tsulukidze et al., 2014).

The value of electronic media is also often overlooked, and some patients are ahead of us in this process. The accessibility of social media means that patients can find out and share information instantly. Reading the blogs of patients with common or rare conditions or from the recently bereaved is chastening. The frankness of these exchanges is often at odds with many of the face-to-face discussions between doctor and patient. Rather than being threatened by these developments, we need to understand why some of our patients can express themselves with devastating frankness online and respond appropriately. There is no reason why many of the questions that cannot be covered at interview, often because of time restrictions or simply the inhibition of the occasion, cannot be answered easily through social media channels. Indeed, often more considered, thoughtful supportive answers can be given, read and re-read by both participants.

BOX 12.7

Read this article: www.theatlantic.com/science/archive/2022/10/five-stages-complicated-grief-wrong/671710/

Death is a sanitised and taboo subject in modern society. We need to reclaim it so that we can all tell our stories. Saul, an intensivist from New Zealand, advises that we all make a plan around death, that we think through the Where, What we want in terms of intervention and Who is going to ensure that our plan is followed. Whoever our advocate is, family member, friend or colleague, they need the time, the proximity and the ability to act under pressure. The question for us all is: If we were unable to speak for ourselves or indicate our wishes, who would know what we wanted and be able to communicate that appropriately?

BOX 12.8 TOOLS FOR REFLECTION

- www.open.edu/openlearn/education/learning-teach-becoming-reflective-practitioner/content-section-6
- www.gponline.com/developing-reflective-writing-skills-part-one/article/1137992
- www.westlakesgptraining.org.uk/pdfs/Reflective%20writing%20guide%20HENE.pdf

BOX 12.9

I find it helps to see life as being like a book: Just as a book is bounded by its covers, by beginning and end, so our lives are bounded by birth and death, and even though a book is limited by beginning and end, it can encompass distant landscapes, exotic figures, fantastic adventures. And even though a book is limited by beginning and end, the characters within it know no horizons. They only know the moments that make up their story, even when the book is closed. And so the characters of a book are not afraid of reaching the last page. Long John Silver is not afraid of you finishing your copy of Treasure Island. And so it should be with us. Imagine the book of your life, its covers, its beginning and end, and your birth and your death. You can only know the moments in between, the moments that make up your life. It makes no sense for you to fear what is outside of those covers, whether before your birth or after your death. And you needn't worry how long the book is, or whether it's a comic strip or an epic. The only thing that matters is that you make it a good story.

(Stephen Cave)

We need to reclaim death as a natural process and take it away from the medicalised world it currently inhabits. We need to remember that increased longevity means increased old age, not increased youth. We can learn much from other disciplines and cultures. We can deny or fail to confront our own mortality, but there is an inescapable truth: life goes on. We are born, live and die, but others – family, friends, colleagues – continue. What we feel, has been experienced by countless generations before. Because of our apparent technological sophistication and belief that science can fix everything, modern mechanisms for coping are, however, perhaps less developed. The early Greek philosophers highlighted the need for *ataraxia* – the equilibrium needed to continue in the face of loss and trauma. As George Bonanno high-lights – we are ultimately resilient. If our lives are our stories, then our deaths must be viewed as part of the narrative. For some, death will represent the end of the book; for others the conclusion of a chapter. However viewed, the story can and should be told – if possible with laughter and compassion.

> *Nobody ever figures out what life is all about, and it doesn't matter. Explore the world. Nearly everything is really interesting if you go into it deeply enough. ... The highest forms of understanding we can achieve are laughter and human compassion.*

(Richard Feynman)

REFERENCES AND FURTHER READING

A Good Death. Time to think. NHS Public Health North East 2010. Available at: www.phine.org.uk/uploads/doc/vid_8535_Full%20report%20with%20all%20appendices.pdf

Brandt H.E., Ooms M.E., Ribbe M.W., van der Wal G., Deliens L. Predicted survival vs. actual survival in terminally ill noncancer patients in Dutch nursing homes. *J. Pain Symptom Manag.* 2006; *32*: 560–6.

Cave S. Available at: https://www.ted.com/talks/stephen_cave_the_4_stories_we_tell_ourselves_about_death?language=en

Chow E., Harth T., Hruby G., Finkelstein J., Wu J., Danjoux C. How accurate are physicians' clinical predictions of survival and the available prognostic tools in estimating survival times in terminally ill cancer patients? A systematic review. *Clin Oncol (R. Coll. Radiol.).* 2001; *13*: 209–18.

Costello J. Dying well: Nurses' experiences of 'good and bad' deaths in hospital. *J. Adv. Nurs.* 2006; *54*: 594–601.

DeJong J.D., Clarke L.E. What is a good death? Stories from palliative care. *J. Palliat. Care* 2009; *25*: 61–7.

Diehl M., Coyle N., Labouvie-Vief G. Age and sex differences in strategies of coping and defense across the life span. *Psychol. and Aging* 1996; *11*: 127–139.

Dying Matters Survey 2014 conducted by ComRes. Available at: www.comres.co.uk/wp-content/themes/comres/poll/NCPC_Dying_Matters_Data_tables.pdf

Elwyn G., Buckman L. Should doctors encourage patients to record consultations? *BMJ.* 2015; *350*: g7645.

Evans D.W., Milanak M.E., Medeiros B., Ross J.L. Magical beliefs and rituals in young children. *Child Psychiatry and Human Development* 2002; *33*: 43–58.

Finlay E., Casarett D. Making difficult discussions easier. *Ca. Cancer J. Clin.* 2009; *59*: 250–63.

First national VOICES survey of bereaved people: Key findings report. Department of Health 2012.

Gorer G. The pornography of death. In: *Death, Grief and Mourning in Contemporary Britain.* London: Cresset; 1955.

Heckhausen J., Schulz R. A life-span theory of control. *Psychol. Rev.* 1995; *102*: 284–304.

Kübler-Ross E. *On death and dying: What the dying have to teach doctors, nurses, clergy and their own families.* Foreword by Byock I Scribner. New York, London, Toronto, Sydney, New Dehli: Scribner Book Company; 2014.

Lawton M.P., Kleban M.H., Dean J. Affect and age: Cross-sectional comparisons of structure and prevalence. *Psychol Aging* 1993; *8*: 165–175.

Leadbetter C., Garber J. *Dying for change.* London: Demos; 2010.

Bolton D. Dearsley P., Madronal-Luque R., Baron-Cohen S. Magical thinking in childhood and adolescence: Development and relation to obsessive compulsion. *British J. Dev. Psychol.* 2002; *20*, 479–94.

Maltoni M., Caraceni A., Brunelli C., et al. Prognostic factors in advanced cancer patients: Evidence-based clinical recommendations – A study by the Steering Committee of the European Association for Palliative Care. *J. Clin Oncol.* 2005 September 1; *23*(25): 6240–8.

Maxfield M., Kluck B., Greenberg J., et al. Age-related differences in responses to thoughts of one's own death: Mortality salience and judgments of moral transgressions. *Psychol. Aging.* 2007; *22*: 341–53.

Mroczek D.K., Kolarz C.M. The effect of age on positive and negative affect: A developmental perspective on happiness. *J. Pers. Soc. Psychol.* 1998; *75*: 1333–1349.

Pocock S.J., Ariti C.A. McMurray J.J.V., et al. Predicting survival in heart failure: A risk score based on 39372 patients from 30 studies. *Eur. Heart J.* 2013; *34*: 1404–13.

Pullman P. *The amber spyglass.* Scholastic, David Fickling Books; 2002.

Romanoff B.D., Thomson B.E. Meaning construction in palliative care: The use of narrative, ritual and the expressive arts. *Am. J. Hospice and Palliative Med.* 2006; *23*: 309–16.

Smith R. Dying of cancer is the best death. Accessed at: http://blogs.bmj.com/bmj/2014/12/31/richard-smith-dying-of-cancer-is-the-best-death/

Smith R. A good death. *British Med. J.* 2000; *320*: 129–30.

Steinhauser K.E., Clipp E.C., McNeilly M., et al. In search of a good death: Observations of patients, families, and providers. *Ann. Intern. Med.* 2000 May 16; *132*: 825–32.

Tsulukidze M., Durand M.-A., Barr P.J., Mead T., Elwyn G. Providing recording of clinical consultations to patients – A highly valued but underutilized intervention: A scoping review. *Patient Educ. Couns.* 2014; *95*: 297–304.

Wollstonecraft M. *Letters written during a short residence in Sweden, Norway and Denmark.* London: Joseph Johnson; 1796.

Woolley J.D. Thinking about fantasy: Are children fundamentally different thinkers and believers from adults? *Child Dev.* 1997; *68*: 991–1011.

INDEX

Printed in the United States
by Baker & Taylor Publisher Services